"Hello, there, Dr. Henry."

And there she was. The woman he'd tried not to think about for far too long. Dressed in a white floating beach dress with a low neckline, a peppermint-beaded necklace nestled against her brown skin between the curve of her breasts. Her blond hair, like spun gold in some fairy tale, hung loose to her shoulders and caught the light from the big windows.

She'd grown even more beautiful and there was an air of confidence and serenity that she hadn't had when he'd first seen her.

His heart went boom and his breath caught. *Nadia Hargraves, be still my heart.*

To his delight she leaned forward and kissed his cheek. Not quite beyond his wildest dreams but pretty darn near it. "That's to say thank you for all the times you reassured me about Katie in the NICU. I don't think I did say thanks."

"You are very welcome." He forced himself to release her hands. Remembered where he was. Who he was. Though he didn't really know who she was now.

Dear Reader,

Welcome back to Rainbow Bay, just below the Gold Coast in Queensland, Australia. Consultant pediatrician Henry Oliver has loved Nadia Hargraves from the first moment he saw her, pushed in a wheelchair to a crib in the NICU, but for four years he's based the picture he's carried in his head on her most difficult time, and the fact his own hardworking mom died young without support.

For Nadia, it was hard work pulling herself out of the shock of widowhood, having a premature baby and paying off unexpected debts, but thanks to family support and determination, she's her own woman now. She isn't going to set herself up for another loss by falling in love and risk losing it all again.

I love introducing two people to each other and watching the fireworks as they push and pull their way to love.

And I always find it fun to return to people (I suppose they're fictional characters but to me they are people) I've known, seen fall in love and begin their lives together. I do hope you enjoy your visit to Rainbow Bay as much as I did, aptly named as a place of hope and new beginnings.

Fiona x

FALLING FOR THE SINGLE MOM NEXT DOOR

FIONA McARTHUR

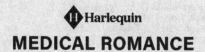

MEDICAL ROMANCE

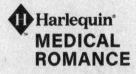

Harlequin®
MEDICAL ROMANCE

ISBN-13: 978-1-335-94284-5

Falling for the Single Mom Next Door

Harlequin Enterprises ULC
22 Adelaide St. West, 41st Floor
Toronto, Ontario M5H 4E3, Canada
www.Harlequin.com

Printed in U.S.A.

Recycling programs
for this product may
not exist in your area.

Fiona McArthur is an Australian midwife who lives in the country and loves to dream. Writing medical romance gives Fiona the chance to write about all the wonderful aspects of romance, adventure, medicine and the midwifery she feels so passionate about. When she's not catching babies, Fiona and her husband, Ian, are off to meet new people, see new places and have wonderful adventures. Drop in and say hi at Fiona's website, fionamcarthurauthor.com.

Books by Fiona McArthur

Harlequin Medical Romance

The Midwives of Lighthouse Bay

A Month to Marry the Midwife
Healed by the Midwife's Kiss
The Midwife's Secret Child

Christmas in Lyrebird Lake

Midwife's Christmas Proposal
Midwife's Mistletoe Baby

Christmas with Her Ex
Second Chance in Barcelona
Taking a Chance on the Best Man
Father for the Midwife's Twins
Healing the Baby Doc's Heart

Visit the Author Profile page
at Harlequin.com for more titles.

Dedicated to my dear friend Tracy Brenton, who
helped me understand Nadia.

**Praise for
Fiona McArthur**

"I absolutely adored the story.... Highly recommended
for fans of contemporary romance. I look forward to
reading more of Fiona McArthur's work."
—*Goodreads* on *Healed by the Midwife's Kiss*

PROLOGUE

Almost five years previously
Henry

DR HENRY OLIVER, paediatric registrar, hadn't thought he would fall for someone at first sight.

Heck, Henry loved the company of women, enjoyed the rapport between colleagues in the hospital and supposed, after careful consideration, he'd one day settle down and have a family with a like-minded partner most probably in the medical profession.

But on this day, at work, his romantic soul felt captured by the mother of a patient—a woman in a wheelchair, as pale as death—so not in his plans. He'd been standing beside a wall, writing notes on his tablet about a tiny prem, unaware that his life was about to change direction.

Henry's boss, Simon Purdy, consultant paediatrician and neonatologist, was the one who pushed the wheelchair towards the open crib and Henry looked up to see the woman's golden hair wisping around her fine-boned cheeks like pale sunrays. The young mother held one delicate hand under her chin as if her head felt too heavy for her slender neck to carry the burden as she gazed upon her child who had been fighting for survival but refused to succumb.

Henry felt as if he'd been blinded by fog his entire life.

The fog instantly dissipated and even from across the room Henry could see the enormous sapphire eyes fill with maternal angst and the sparkle of unshed tears as she lifted her chin to Simon. Henry needed to be there for her.

She was a patient's mother, yet without even noticing his presence he felt her call to him. An unexpected wave of protectiveness tightened his chest and Henry reached out to touch the wall to steady himself. His body went cold and then heated. He had never had such feelings before, except perhaps as a young boy when his single mother had worked too hard. He'd wanted to nurture and protect her like this, and had failed. But this woman was not his responsibility.

At least he was older. Wiser. Not a child. He knew from Simon that this woman was a recent widow and was surrounded by family and grieving—nowhere near being emotionally available.

No room for him to be more to her—possibly for years.

This feeling of recognition was crazy, unexpected, but it seemed to hold such significance he couldn't brush it away.

Thank goodness he was leaving soon for London, but still his eyes fixed on the angel in the blue dressing gown, confirming who she was, her premature baby and her scarily efficient sister, intensivist Isabella Hargraves. And Simon, his senior consultant, who was his boss and her baby's doctor. But he'd never actually seen *Nadia* until now and that must be why his world had tilted.

Over the next four weeks, before Henry left for the new appointment in London, he made himself available to Nadia when she needed extra support, not pushing, answering her hundreds of questions as her baby grew, staying quietly in the background, and acknowledged ruefully that he wasn't visible to her even though she felt seared into his heart.

Strangely, the crazy concept didn't rattle him. He had nothing to offer her at this time and she was grieving. Immersed in the needs of her tiny daughter. Lost in being a widow and single parent. Surrounded by her family. He was invisible.

Lucky he was going, it really was, because here there was only heartache for him.

Almost five years later

Dr Henry Oliver signed on the dotted line and the pretty redheaded Realtor sat back and fluttered her extra-long eyelashes in an I-could-give-you-more-than-legal-papers-if-you-want look.

In London, Marco, his ex-flatmate, certainly would have been eager to secure a phone number.

Not Henry. Not now. Not on the Gold Coast back in Australia.

This was the real world and he'd be too busy at work for romance in the next year or two.

Henry felt delighted about the signing but not tempted by the pretty girl. He'd just bought his favourite apartment, ocean view overlooking Rainbow Bay, Queensland, top floor, in a small block of units that each took up the whole floor. He'd always loved this apartment.

Though he believed it was good business sense, even if it had cost a packet, he couldn't help but wonder how much of this decision was tied to the woman who, he'd just discovered, still lived downstairs.

No. He'd bought the place because he'd always fancied it when he came to visit his boss, Simon, when he'd worked for him as a registrar. The hospital where he'd be spending a lot of time working was one street away and Simon's partnership in his thriving Gold Coast paediatric practice was not much further to walk.

It just felt so good to be back in Australia after years at London's GOSH, the Great Ormond Street Hospital for Children, though he had thrived working in paediatrics under leaders in the field. His work and living away from Oz had been exhausting, though Marco had made it fun.

Henry had flat shared with an Italian colleague, Marco, who pushed weights in his off time and dragged Henry with him to the gym until Henry had never been so fit or confident in himself.

Henry enjoyed the company of women but, apart from forced double dates with his flatmate's latest girlfriend's girlfriend, he rarely thought of anything but work.

Now, back in Australia, he'd achieved the professional goal of paediatric consultant he'd always dreamed of becoming while still being one of the younger specialists at thirty-four.

And then his boss—no, his colleague—Simon had oh-so-casually mentioned that his sister-in-law Nadia was still single.

Henry's heart quickened, but that was because of his purchase—heck, he'd always loved Simon's home. Nothing to do with Nadia.

Yes. He'd bought the place because he loved the apartment.

None of that decision had been tied to the single mother who lived downstairs.

Nothing to do with Nadia.

CHAPTER ONE

Nadia

NADIA HARGRAVES PUSHED the base of the child's swing harder and Katie, a very mature almost five-year-old, giggled in the strapped swing seat.

'Push me higher, Mummy.'

Nadia watched the mane of her daughter's blonde hair streaming in the wind as they both faced out over the waves and across the bay to Surfers Paradise with each push.

On their side of the water, the white sand of Rainbow Bay, so aptly named as a place of hope and new beginnings, stretched to the break wall where the waves crashed and creamed up the side of the jagged rocks. Every now and then a larger set of waves would shoot droplets into the sky with a snap and a fan of crystal water. Ahead, surfers swooped forwards or slid backwards off waves, while seagulls cawed above.

Here was so much better than Sydney's snarling traffic or Brisbane's constant roadworks. This tucked-away southern corner of the Gold Coast had become Nadia's favourite place in the world.

Here she had her daughter Katie, her only sister Bella, plus, of course, Bella's caring husband Simon and their son Kai and her grandmother Catherine, all close in one apartment block—and they were the most important people in her world.

Occasionally her professor father visited briefly from Sydney if he had a business appointment in the Gold Coast, but years of work-related neglect from him meant none of the women in his life had expectations of a lasting connection. Even for his favourite, Isabella, Dad could easily visit the hospital next door and not even consider calling in to see his grandchildren before he flew way again.

Nadia had learnt in childhood that she could survive without her father, any man really, in her life. Until she'd fallen for Alex. But he was gone. Wrapping his expensive new car around a telegraph pole and leaving her just enough of her own savings to buy the apartment outright and barely any savings to survive on. She'd managed to navigate pregnancy, widowhood, moving, a difficult birth and motherhood without Alex.

Maybe because as a young girl her famous father had always loved his work more than his two motherless daughters, she'd understood that for Alex she'd taken second place as well.

The number of times she'd watched fruitlessly

for Dad to arrive at childhood occasions and been disappointed. Birthdays, awards, graduations, he hadn't come to any. Piers Hargraves had taught Nadia well that complete immersion in work was a bad thing, so marrying a doctor had been out. Her dear old dad might be an expert neurologist in Sydney, but he knew little of the caring side of his brain and Nadia had finally given up trying for his approval. Even when she'd voiced her dream of being a nurse like Bella, more for him than herself she suspected now, hadn't made him see her.

But she'd fallen for her handsome husband, had thought easy-going Alex was the answer, but that hadn't worked out either. He'd been too busy socialising to be there for her, despite taking her surname when they'd married. Nadia had secretly questioned whether he'd hoped to become the favoured son-in-law and benefit financially from her dad.

Poor Alex had turned out to be less than perfect, uninvested in anyone apart from himself, and had left her an impoverished widow when he'd wrapped one of his fast cars around a pole a few months before their daughter had been born.

But she had loved him, although she'd been disappointed by who she thought he was when he'd died, until the reality of the financial disasters he'd wrought in so short a time had become apparent and she'd had to climb out of a financial hole.

The drone of a plane rose above the din of the surf for a moment, interrupting her thoughts, and as its wings came in low to disappear behind the hill of apartments to her left to land at the hidden airport, Nadia remembered her broken arrival that fateful year.

Refuge in Gran's apartment had saved her, and then using her savings to make her own home in Gran's block.

She'd been pregnant and shell-shocked at the loss, but Gran and her sister had steered her safely to finding her feet in the spacious ground floor unit near family.

Best move ever.

'Ahoy, you two,' a familiar voice called out. And here came the dearest member of her family now.

Her sister Isabella, tall, blonde and very pregnant, strode, only slightly ungainly despite her huge baby bump, across the grass towards them. Nadia shook her head in admiration. Nothing slowed Bella down. Not even a watermelon-sized belly.

Nadia let go of the swing and reached out to hug her sibling, the big bulge in the way making her smile widen. 'How on earth can you still move so fast? It defies mechanical physics.'

Bella shrugged. 'Women are designed to be adjustable when pregnant.' She waved at her niece. 'Hello, darling Katie.'

'Hello, Auntie Bella.' Katie blew a kiss, then set her chin and began to lean forward and backward, trying to get the swing to increase momentum on her own, while her mother stood distracted.

Bella rubbed her hands. 'Guess what!'

Nadia steeled herself for what she suspected might be coming. 'What?'

'We sold the unit.'

Nadia's heart sank and she tried not to let disappointment show. Bella was moving out. 'That's great news for you all. Yay. Simon will be happy.'

She could see that, uncharacteristically, Bella was oblivious of her sense of impending loss. She must be very excited because her sister rarely missed anything.

Bella burbled on, 'Kai will be so happy. He can learn to ride a pushbike in his own backyard. I'll have space for baby and spare rooms as well.' She laughed. 'Several rooms. It's a big house.'

'And you'll have areas for entertaining.' She knew Bella and her friends were multiplying children and the unit was proving too small for social events. 'The buyer must have snapped it up as this is the first I've heard.'

'He did. But then he'd seen the place years ago. Do you remember Henry Oliver, Simon's registrar from when Katie was born?'

Henry Oliver? On hearing his name, Nadia found it surprisingly easy to conjure kind brown eyes and very short brown hair. Henry Oliver. Good grief. She'd liked Henry. A tall but slim man with a diffident manner and the nicest smile. 'Yes. I do remember Henry.'

He'd been so attentive, caring and thoughtful of her feelings. Unlike Alex. Where had that thought come from?

She steered her thoughts away. 'Didn't you take him under your wing and teach him some tricks for difficult cannulas?'

'Good grief, I'd forgotten that.' Bella laughed. 'I was feeling protective of Katie, and you weren't there.'

No. She hadn't been there when her precious daughter had been admitted to the NICU at thirty-two weeks. And her husband had been dead. She'd been in Intensive Care with severe hypertension of pregnancy, fighting for her life, while her prem daughter had been watched over by her fierce neonatal nurse aunt Bella.

Nadia whispered, 'I'm fairly sure you told Henry he wasn't allowed to attempt to cannulate my baby again until you gave him some lessons.' She was teasing but even the memory made her want to hug her sister.

Bella nodded, a little pink in the cheeks. 'It was four a.m. I wasn't allowed to treat a relative, so I made him ring Simon to come in.'

'That's when you fell in love with Simon.'

'Not that night,' Bella said with a laugh. 'But soon after.'

Her sister and brother-in-law were a besotted couple and their love gave her hope for some distant time in the future.

'I remember Henry told me you terrified him.' Nadia laughed at her sister's expression. 'You do get scary when you're in NICU.'

Bella couldn't help being an extremely skilled nurse when she wasn't on maternity leave. As their father still said, she should have been a doctor. But Bella loved hands-on paediatric intensive care and had no desire to work in medical rooms half the time seeing patients.

Bella laughed. 'Oh, piffle. But you'd better not remind him I was pushy because he's joined Simon's practice as a consulting partner and coming to work at our hospital.'

For some reason Nadia doubted the Henry she had memories of would hold a grudge. He hadn't seemed that type of person.

She felt a flash of delight at the news. Probably because she now knew there wouldn't be strangers in the top unit. He'd been good to her when he'd been the neonatal registrar, when Simon or her sister had been busy elsewhere, and Henry had always eased her worries when she had something on her mind.

Yes, Henry had helped her understand about prematurity and the temporary heart murmur

they'd found in Katie, and all the other things a
newly widowed mother would worry about with
her prem baby. Yes. He'd been very kind.

She wondered if she'd ever thanked him.

CHAPTER TWO

Henry

HENRY HAD ALWAYS been methodical, perhaps stemming from when he'd hunkered down and tried everything he could to not be a burden on his hardworking mother. If he wanted something he worked steadily towards his goal, using his own tenacious resolve to achieve said objective. A year or two of knuckled-down hard work and he'd achieve all he wanted here too.

In the last three days Henry had accomplished a lot. He had furniture ready to go into the apartment when he took possession. He'd settled into the specialist practice he'd bought into. And he'd acquired his own residents, Tom and Sam, and Amelia, a brilliant and careful registrar, to share the workload and create his team.

He'd taken on the hospital consultant paediatric position for both the Emergency Department and Children's Ward, quite a workload, when he started at the hospital next week.

Rainbow Bay Hospital had proved not as large or imposing as London experience had taught him to expect, but he preferred the modern and more patient-centric model, with hopefully more time to get to know patients and parents.

His new office with its large windows looking over Coolangatta Beach showcased everything he'd missed about living in Australia. Blue skies, sparkling ocean, a laid-back but surprisingly efficient secretary of his own, and a stellar senior partner to forge ahead with in his professional life. Hard to believe it was the Friday of his first week because he felt as if he was finally home.

Right now, after work, Henry carried a bottle of Tasmanian Coal River Pinot Noir, a red wine he'd missed and aspired to open. He straightened his tie with his other hand as he stepped out of the lift, casting slightly proprietorial eyes around the foyer outside his soon-to-be front door.

He'd been looking forward to Simon and Isabella's farewell party in the flat and been invited to come early. In fact, he'd spent far too much time today anticipating the moment he arrived.

Because tonight he would see Nadia Hargraves. He hadn't caught a glimpse of her for almost five years. There was no doubt that she had been on his mind but he'd probably blown the whole attraction-at-first-sight thing out of proportion. Most likely, it had just been a protective instinct since he'd known her circumstances.

Anyway, he'd also see Nadia's daughter, Katie. He couldn't imagine that tiny, thirty-two-week baby as almost five years old. Of course, for a paediatrician there was nothing more satisfying to see than a struggling baby become a healthy and happy child. Nadia's child.

He knocked, and after some delay the door opened slowly to reveal a waist-high, woebegone blonde-haired little girl with two big tears sliding down her pink cheeks. She looked healthy but not a happy child. Despite the mermaid suit.

The tiny mermaid sniffed and rubbed the back of her hand under her nose. He glanced behind her but there were no adults that he could see. Odd? But kids didn't faze Henry. He enjoyed and admired children. Spent his days with them.

He tilted his head, crouched down and said, 'Hello. I'm Dr Henry. What's wrong, sweetheart?' He pulled out the large white handkerchief he always carried and dabbed her cheeks, then handed it to her. 'Blow.'

She took it and with a surprisingly vigorous trumpet she blew, and he couldn't help but smile.

'Better,' he said, taking the screwed ball of his handkerchief back carefully to keep his hands clean and tucking it into his trouser pocket to sanitise later. 'Now, tell me what's made you feel sad.'

'Mummy and Auntie Bella are dressing Kai, and I was feeding Ernestine…' She stopped. Held up a much-loved rag doll.

'Something happened?' Henry glanced around the room until he saw. Under one of the low tables a tipped plate of biscuits and several rounds of cheese had ended up in a scatter of food and crackers on the pristine tiled floor. 'Did your doll bump the plate?'

Another sniff. A nod. And big beautiful green eyes swam with tears again.

Henry stood up. Held out his hand. 'Oh, no, you don't. We'll just fix the plate, and you and your doll will say sorry to Auntie Bella and Mummy, and everyone will be happy. Okay?'

'You sure?'

'It's not a big thing. And we can fix it. Lickety-split.'

The little girl blinked and lifted her chin. 'I'm Katie.'

'I thought you might be. I met you when you were a tiny baby. You're a big girl now.'

'I am.'

They crossed to the scene of the accident and Henry used a biscuit to push the cheeses back onto the plate and into some semblance of attractive arrangement while Katie picked up the biscuits. 'Are there more biscuits in the kitchen?'

Katie nodded.

'Let's put these ones in the bin and put out new ones when you wash your hands.'

When Katie frowned at him he added, 'I don't think Auntie Bella would mind.'

'Hello, Henry.' His new partner's wife gave him one of her warm smiles as she walked in. She was wearing a tent. It was a very pretty tent, but my goodness she was pregnant, Henry thought in some awe.

She raised her brows at her niece. 'What wouldn't Auntie Bella mind?'

Isabella glanced at the biscuits in Katie's hands and the one in Simon's and smiled. 'Ah, I see. The cheese fell. And we need new biscuits. I don't mind at all.' She stepped forward with her hand out. 'Let me take that plate.'

'I have to wash my hands.' Katie waved them in the air. 'Dr Henry said.'

Another movement from the bedrooms. 'Hello there, Dr Henry.'

And there she was. The woman he'd tried not to think about for far too long. Dressed in a floating white beach dress with a low neckline, a peppermint beaded necklace nestled against her brown skin between the curve of her breasts. Her blonde hair, like spun gold in some fairy tale, hung loose to her shoulders and caught the light from the big windows.

She'd grown even more beautiful and there was an air of confidence and serenity that she hadn't had when he'd first seen her.

His heart went boom and his breath caught. *Nadia Hargraves...be still my heart.*

The seconds seemed to stretch as his gaze

snagged on the woman he suddenly realised he'd measured every other female in London against, finding they fell short. He'd been an idiot.

He stepped forward. An idiot with great taste. The rest of the room was forgotten.

His hands stretched out to take hers. 'Nadia.'

The word was a breath as he captured her slim fingers, her skin as warm and soft and exquisite as he'd imagined it would feel beneath his. If he'd thought before that he'd come home... For one crazy moment he believed he really breathed *home*—which was ridiculous. They were practically strangers.

To his delight, she leaned forward and kissed his cheek. Not quite beyond his wildest dreams but pretty darn near it. 'That's to say thank you for all the times you reassured me about Katie in the NICU. I don't think I did say thanks.'

'You are very welcome.' He forced himself to release her hands. Remembered where he was. Who he was. Though he didn't really know who she was now.

He turned back to the others, who were watching. 'And Katie has grown up to be a beauty like her mother.' He smiled. 'And her aunt.' He needed some sanity. 'Where's Simon?'

He noted that Isabella watched them both with a definite twinkle in her eyes so like her sister's, though she glanced at the door. 'He was called back to the unit but shouldn't be long. He's been gone an hour already.'

At that moment a key turned in the lock and the door swung open. 'Perfect timing,' his wife said as Dr Simon Purdy, tall, debonair, greying a little at the temples and Henry's senior partner, entered the room.

'Uncle Simon—' Katie grabbed Henry's hand and pulled him towards the door '—this is Dr Henry.'

Everyone laughed and poor Katie frowned as Henry gently squeezed her tiny hand and crouched down. 'You didn't know but Uncle Simon and I have known each other for a long time. But thank you, it was very kind of you to introduce me. Did Mummy tell you that I'll be moving into this flat when your auntie Bella and uncle Simon move to their new house?'

She turned to her mother. 'Is that true?'

'It is,' Nadia confirmed.

'That's nice,' said Katie, shrugging off her confusion. 'We'll be able to come up and visit, just like we do with Auntie Bella.'

Henry stifled a laugh and looked innocently up at Nadia. 'You and Mummy are welcome at any time.'

Nadia murmured, 'Oh, please, don't tell her that,' but the awkward moment passed as the doorbell rang.

Simon opened it to a dark-haired man and his

blonde wife, their tow-headed twins and one dark-haired baby.

Henry knew Malachi Madden and his wife Lisandra and their two little boys. His eyes widened. 'My goodness, look at your boys, Malachi.'

He smiled at Lisandra, a woman he admired very much, and shook hands with Malachi. Lisandra leaned in and kissed his cheek. He hadn't met the baby in Lisandra's arms. 'And who is this little pearl?'

'This is Angelica. She's eight weeks old today.'

Katie's little voice said, 'You really do know almost everybody.'

'I know these people,' Henry said as he smiled down at her. 'And these boys, though they were only slightly bigger than you were when I left.'

'We're at school now,' Bastian said. 'But Bennett's not in my class.' He sounded miffed.

The boys weren't shy then.

Henry said sagely, 'I heard they do that with twins.'

CHAPTER THREE

Nadia

NADIA WATCHED HENRY assimilate into the close group with ridiculous ease—not the quiet, diffident man she remembered but a man who stood out even in this crowd of men who shone. This version of Henry Oliver seemed larger than life.

Way larger than life. Good grief, no diffidence here, just confidence, and those shoulders and arms—he could lift her up and toss her over his shoulder without breathing hard. Now why on earth had she thought of that? But she couldn't help the smile at the ridiculous picture.

As if echoing her thoughts, the latest man to arrive, and her own obstetrician, Malachi Madden, spoke up bluntly as usual. 'What happened to you, Henry—take up bodybuilding in London? You're twice the size you were!'

'A bit of exaggeration there, Malachi.' Henry laughed and the deep, rumbling sound rolled over her, tingling her skin. 'Flat-shared with a paed from Italy and we stayed fit at the gym. Had to because it felt like we spent twenty hours a day at the hospital.'

Nadia frowned as she heard that and thought to herself, *Twenty hours a day at the hospital? Good grief. Men. Just like her father.* She mentally nudged away any thoughts of being attracted to Henry. *Shame, that.*

'Maybe I could go run with you here?' Henry said to Malachi. 'I'm a social animal. I like company when I exercise.'

Malachi grinned. 'You can try to catch me.'

'Or not.' The men sized each other up with amusement. 'A race never bothered me.'

Nadia decided that Henry didn't look worried or hang back from being competitive. He really was not the Henry she remembered. And that was enough thinking about Henry. She wasn't the woman he remembered either, she imagined.

'No running on Saturdays,' Isabella stated. 'Lisandra comes surfing with us. We go every week while the men mind the children.'

Simon touched his niece's blonde head. 'And Katie's a big help when I mind Kai, aren't you, sweetheart?'

Katie nodded importantly.

'I might have to take up surfing myself.' Henry's gaze shifted from Katie to her, a brush of teasing, and Nadia felt it as if he'd lifted his finger to her cheek. Why was he looking at her when he said that? She wasn't surfing with him.

She did not want a man in her life, or if she ever did… It wouldn't be a career consultant like her father.

Oh, boy, no.

Henry Oliver had just admitted that he lived and breathed the hospital and buried himself in work. Even worse, she didn't need another man who would draw the eye of every woman he passed like her departed husband had. And there was no doubt that this new Henry would do that too.

Henry tilted his head when she didn't answer. There was a smile on his face, darn it, a really too handsome face, waiting for her to smile back. 'You surf too, Nadia?'

The doorbell rang again.

She lifted her chin. 'Bella and I surfed for years. Our gran was one of the original Bondi Girls and she taught us both. Gran was a champion.'

Simon ushered in Catherine, speak of the dear devil, just as she uttered that. Nadia saw that Elsa Green, the lady from two floors down, was with her, along with her visiting granddaughter, Lisa, whose eyes jumped straight to Henry with speculation. Really? Lisa was just going to stare at him with big eyes?

She heard Gran say sedately, 'Did I hear my name?'

'We were talking about surfing,' Bella said. 'So of course your name came up.'

There was a general surge of people hugging and kissing and suddenly it was crowded with nine adults, three children, a baby and an enormous pregnant belly in the unit.

Nadia stepped back and away and Henry moved with her, saying from her other side, 'I think, yes, your sister needs a bigger house.'

Nadia had to laugh. 'Despite my loss. I fear so.' She looked at him then while the others exchanged pleasantries. 'Are you excited about moving in?'

He took in the layout of the apartment and she studied him while his attention was focused on the room around them. Sexy, confident, muscular, gorgeous—not descriptions she would have thought of for the old Henry, which was strange—but certainly fitting now. And in this setting, with people she knew so well, it was surprising that he looked so very much at home.

'It's great to be back,' he murmured. His eyes sparkled as he looked over his shoulder at her. 'And yes, I've always loved the view from this unit.' He gestured with his arm to the small balcony, inviting her to step out there with him.

She didn't know why but she followed him, leaning her elbows on the rail and turning her face to watch his expression as he leaned his strong arms on the warm metal.

'I love the ocean. The colours. All of it. When Simon said he was selling I decided to go for this.'

She thought about that. About what she knew of him, which wasn't much except he'd been good to her and Katie in the past. And now he'd come back a very well-built paediatric consultant working with her brother-in-law—no doubt after long hours of intense medicine and loads of experience.

She thought again of his care of Katie. 'I'm glad. You work hard and deserve a place you can relax in.' That was true. He'd been incredibly knowledgeable five years ago. He'd be more so now. The hospital was lucky to have him back. And now he was Simon's partner, she guessed, she'd see a lot of him.

She thought about that and a strange, agitated feeling grew inside her, but her expression must have stayed the same because he only said, 'Thank you. I appreciate that.'

'Anyone special in your life to share your view?' Now why had she asked that? Good grief. Her eye caught on Lisa, watching them through the glass. You'd think she'd pretend she wasn't watching Henry. Nadia looked away. And why did she care?

His teeth flashed in a quick white grin. 'Not yet. Currently, I'm footloose and fancy-free.'

At the wattage of his smile her attention zeroed in on him. 'Hardly footloose, buying into Simon's

practice and working at the hospital all hours.
What about your parents? Siblings?'

'No family.' The smile died and there was
something quiet in his tone that didn't match the
man, the view or the conversation. He directed
the topic away from himself. 'Do you still enjoy
living here?'

No family? Curiosity stirred and she tamped
it down. Then frowned at herself. She shouldn't
even have started asking questions. Let it go.

She remembered he'd asked a question. 'Here?
Good grief, I love the place.' Glad to change the
subject with him.

She gestured with her hand at the park below
and the expanse of water around them. 'This is
my world. I'm in charge. I'm in control.' She heard
the words, the assertion—she'd said that almost
defiantly. It was true but… Good grief. Talk about
putting it out there and waving it like a flag.

His eyes twinkled. 'Sounds like a castle with
a moat.'

Her cheeks felt warm. 'It does.' And maybe that
was too stark for this conversation too.

She relaxed her shoulders and glanced back inside. 'I'll miss having Bella upstairs, but Gran is
still here, and we'll all visit her. And Katie loves
the park. And the beach.'

'When does Katie start school?'

'It's Queensland, so she'll start prep school this
year because she turns five before the thirtieth of

June. She's in childcare now. They don't call it kindergarten up here and it's not compulsory but I work two days a week. I think she should get used to school rules.'

'So proper school next year?'

'She says she wants to stay home with me for another year.'

'Tricky.' He smiled. 'I bet you've worked something out.'

'I have.' She smiled back. 'I bought her a surfboard for Christmas and promised to start teaching her on the weekends once she's big enough for Prep.'

He looked mischievous for a few beats, as if not sure how she'd take his next words. 'Maybe you could teach me to surf at the same time? I'm serious about learning.'

Oh, yeah. She could just see that. This big, well-muscled guy, wobbling on a board, all bare skin and sex appeal. While she was supposed to be watching her daughter. Not on your nelly.

'It's the Gold Coast. You have the means. You can pay a surf instructor.'

'You wound me.'

She huffed out a laugh. She enjoyed this sparring too much. 'I doubt that. After years in London staying warm, I imagine your skin is thicker than it looks.'

'It is. But… Wowser. Where's the fun in that?'

'Tough luck.' She glanced back inside. Away

from those laughing liquid eyes. Found Lisa's still on Henry. Frowned. 'Food's on. Better go help in the kitchen.'

CHAPTER FOUR

Henry

HENRY WATCHED HER walk away. Blonde, beautiful and swaying like a gorgeous golden sunflower in the light sea breeze. He'd done that before—watched her walk away, just before he'd left for London, but this time maybe they could be on an equal footing. Nadia was not his patient's mother. 'You've been away nearly five years. No rush, Henry,' he murmured to himself.

He'd taken himself to London and Great Ormond Street Hospital without making plans for the future.

Now he was back, a consultant in his own right, and he found himself far too delighted that Nadia was still single, and even more dazzling in his eyes. Not only that, she and her daughter lived just downstairs from his new penthouse, so there would be chance encounters apart from socialising with the Purdys and the Maddens.

He had some serious thinking to do and this

time she wasn't a grieving widow he had to walk away from. Now, Nadia was an independent woman, in charge and in control of her world. Her words.

He smiled. He liked that in a woman, in Nadia, but hopefully there was room for him somewhere in her world too.

Simon appeared beside him. 'You're not checking out my sister-in-law, are you, Henry?'

Henry dragged his gaze away from Nadia's back to his new partner, who'd appeared at the door. 'Maybe.'

'I did wonder if that was always the plan,' Simon said, a gleam in his eyes. 'But you were away for a long time... I thought I had it wrong.'

Henry shrugged. He'd been determined to come back a success.

'I enjoyed London, enjoyed the experience gained with great mentors. Stepping more into paediatrics than neonatal suits me.'

Simon nodded. 'It's a good move. Works well for our practice to have both covered.' Simon's eyes twinkled. 'Did you know that Nadia works as admin in our children's ward?'

Henry stared in delight. 'You're kidding me.'

'Nope. Wouldn't kid about that. She works Mondays and Tuesdays. With the possibility of an increase when Katie goes to Prep full-time.'

'Now, that is interesting news.' He wouldn't have to keep thinking of ways to run into Nadia.

'I thought it might be.' Simon glanced back inside. 'My wife is waving us back to the party.

Henry grinned and preceded Simon into the warm and noisy room.

Suddenly he was surrounded by family and friends—an unexpected feeling and something he hadn't felt since his alcoholic father had deserted his mother when he was seven.

Henry pulled his thoughts away from the dark times, the times he'd hidden behind his quiet façade and pushed himself to learn everything he could to help, the times he'd watched his proud mother work too hard to keep them fed and housed because she refused any help.

It was too late to save Sara Oliver now, his mother's heart had given out at fifty, but Henry's future wife and children would never be reduced to that penury, and he'd set himself to make a solid foundation that would never leave anyone needy.

But he'd been away a long time and it was nice to feel included here. He'd enjoyed London, although he'd missed Australia, but Marco had been distracting and a good friend. He'd also seemed to have no extended family—which was strange for an Italian—but Marco had never talked about his family either.

Heck, there'd never been anything that wasn't testosterone driven with his Italian flatmate. Transitory girls, gym competitions and long hours at work. The years had flown as he'd raced towards his goal.

And now he was back, he owned an apartment, and was more than ready to take on the world saving sick children.

He might not be ready just yet to settle down with a woman and spend the rest of his life with her, but some down time with Nadia did feel more promising than he'd expected. Now he had to find out if Nadia thought that a good plan.

CHAPTER FIVE

Nadia

MONDAYS WERE ALWAYS a struggle. Katie didn't like Mondays, which put a bit of a dampener on them for Nadia as well.

She understood that while her daughter enjoyed being with the other children at childcare, she would very much prefer to be home with her mother every day. Well, she was home with her four out of seven days.

Nadia had wanted to spend as much time as she could with her workaholic dad after their mother died, but she had received even less attention than Bella—though Bella had always been like a surrogate mother for Nadia to make up for it.

The real *world* meant Nadia needed to work at least part-time, and Katie needed to understand that, because she wanted her daughter to grow up independent and self-sufficient.

But, unlike when her dad had been tasked to pick the girls up from school or events, Nadia made sure she *always* arrived. Usually before the rest of the parents at preschool.

On Mondays and Tuesdays Katie went to childcare, and Nadia jammed in two days of children's ward admin, which she loved despite the busyness. It paid the bills while her photography business paid the extras and built up her savings, which had taken such a beating by her husband. She'd never rely on a man or be left in debt like she had been when Alex had died.

Her friend Carmen, another widow, worked the other three days and was flexible with extra work, so if either of their children were sick, the other had cover.

Carmen's little boy went to preschool with Katie, so both were at ease in the other mother's care. Other days, Gran or Bella could care for Katie if needed. But it was rarely needed.

Yes. Her world worked well. And nobody let her down.

The children's ward had recently been upgraded, with everything made modern, and the caring staff, including Nadia, were delighted with the new furnishings.

This morning when Nadia walked in there was a subdued hint of excitement in the air because today they had a new paediatrician starting and everyone wanted to meet him.

Henry Oliver. In her ward. Nadia couldn't get her brain to sit right with that concept. Simon had told her after the party, and she wondered why Henry hadn't mentioned he'd be the new children's ward consultant.

She supposed he hadn't known she worked here.

Their last boss, Dr Steel, had been a gruff, intelligent and caring man, but with little sense of humour. He'd suddenly retired with an unknown illness. Dr Steel had liked children well enough but had always talked down to them.

Somehow, Nadia knew that wouldn't be Henry's style. The idea made her smile. He'd been marvellous with Katie at the party on Friday afternoon and their children's ward just might get a lift it didn't expect.

She'd almost had to run to get here on time this morning, so unusual for her, until finally Katie had called, 'Come on, Mummy, we'll be late.' Dithering with her hair wasn't her usual style, but this morning…

Digital clocks had a lot to answer for, Nadia thought, stowing her bag in the drawer. When she'd been four, she hadn't been able to read a clock face and tell an adult they were late.

But her hair had been a mission. Normally, she just brushed it out but, for some silly reason, today she'd decided to straighten the ends. And it just hadn't hung right. Now, she feared, it looked like a toilet brush.

A shadow fell across her desk. A tall, well-built shadow.

'Good morning, Nadia.' The deep voice and blinding smile hit her. 'Wow. Your hair looks amazing this morning.'

Fighting the blush and borderline annoyed with herself for such a girlie action, she gathered her wits before she looked up. Suddenly, she realised why she'd been so fiddly. Good grief, she'd done it for Henry. No!

Henry stood just a little back from her desk, as though he wanted to take in the whole picture, ridiculous thought, and it looked like he'd taken pains with his appearance too.

Her brows rose in amusement, and appreciation at the panda bear tie covering the buttons of his well-pressed shirt. A shirt that moulded his shoulders and chest as if it had been made for him. Maybe it had—what did she know? This was a new Henry. A pretty darned fabulous Henry. So much so she needed barriers against all that charm because she was an independent woman, not a fool to drool.

She realised he was waiting for her to answer. 'Oh. Good morning, Dr Oliver.' She stood. 'I'll just take you over to Sister Taylor. She's been waiting for you.'

'Formal,' he murmured for her ears only and smiled. 'It's great to see you here. And I look forward to meeting everyone.'

Tara Taylor was in her office, already rising from the chair behind her desk. Nadia gestured with her hand. 'There she is. I'll leave you in her capable hands.'

'Thank you, Nadia.'

Tara, a tall brunette with red highlights and a big smile, tilted her glossy head at Nadia as if to say, *Do you know him?*

Nadia felt her cheeks warm. 'Dr Oliver was a registrar when Katie was in NICU as a baby.' She smiled at Henry. And yes, he'd been great. Just the thought of those days had her softening her awkwardly stilted attitude towards him. 'He's very patient with explaining things.'

Tara smiled at Henry with approval. 'That's lovely. The parents will appreciate that. Welcome to our ward, Dr Oliver. We're very excited to have our own consultant again. We've been struggling with locums.'

Nadia stepped back and away and returned to her desk, where she had a clear view of Henry charming Tara into a laugh. Tara charmed right back. Oh, goodie. She'd get to watch flirting. Not. And where was all this dog in a manger stuff coming from?

Tara and Henry disappeared into a room where Nadia knew a child had not been recovering as fast as everyone had hoped.

Henry stayed in the room for a long time while Tara came and went with trolleys and IV poles and several trips to the medication room, until finally the door opened and Henry emerged with the child's mother.

'I think Joseph will improve more rapidly now, Dawn. But I'll come back at lunchtime and check on his progress.' From her vantage point near the exit to the ward, Nadia watched the worry recede from the mother's drawn face with his promise.

'Thank you, Doctor.'

Henry the doctor. He was invested. She remembered that from when Katie was born. At least that hadn't changed.

Then Henry was off again to walk around the ward properly, making sure each child knew he had time for them and their parents before he left. There were a lot of laughs and smiles from the staff and even the children seemed brighter by the time Henry had finished his ward round.

She heard him say, 'When I come back after lunch, I'll look for those results coming for Anna, Tara. Let's see if we can get her home.'

'Thank you, Henry, that would be great.'

Seemed everyone was on a first name basis after one visit. Dr Steel wouldn't have been happy, and Nadia smiled down at her keyboard.

'See you later, Nadia.' Henry lifted one hand as he passed her desk, and she lifted her face and met his smile.

'Bye-bye.' Oh, good grief. *Bye-bye?* Too late to suck the words back in. Was she four? She'd been a toddler's mother too long and now she spoke like one.

Henry grinned and kept his hand still while he waved his fingers up and down—just like Katie did. She shook her head and went back to work. The guy was a flirt with everyone, not just her, and just because of their previous friendship she wasn't going to be one of his conquests.

Though maybe she needed instructions for building that Henry barrier. Because that was a spectacular smile he'd just sent her, and like everyone else in the ward she'd felt special too.

Apparently, Henry came and went while she was at lunch, but while she was packing up to go home he returned and appeared beside her desk, where she'd been preparing the next week's theatre list patient files.

'Have a good day, Nadia?'

She tilted her head sideways and met his warm brown gaze. He was flirting again. Her newly constructed forcefield went up with only a little delay.

'Hello, Henry. Yes, thanks. And how was your first day?'

He looked across at the nurses' station. 'Great. It's a well-run ward and the staff are very friendly.'

With your winning ways, I bet they are. Now that had been a snarky thought, and she suspected he didn't deserve it. Protection, Nadia, not snarky, she chastised herself.

'I'm glad.' It was the truth.

'Are you going to get Katie now?'

She wondered why he'd asked. 'Yes. Monday is shopping day, and she likes that. I needed something to help get her over the Monday blues.'

His head bobbed once. 'She has Mummy-going-to-work blues, does she?'

He understood, then.

'Yes. Tough love to leave her two days a week.'

'Two seems very reasonable in this day and age. Kids adjust. It's amazing what they'll adapt to.'

'Actually, three. I have Thursdays on my own at home.'

She was thinking there was something there, a shadow of the past in his eyes, something she hoped he'd share...but he didn't.

'Enjoy shopping,' he said instead and walked past her into the ward.

She might have barriers up against Dr Henry Oliver, but just maybe the intriguing man had a few brick walls of his own to keep out the world.

On Tuesday Henry's spectacular smile seemed a little dimmer as he went past her desk. 'Good morning, Nadia,' he said as he paused.

'Good morning, Henry. Nice bags under your eyes.'

'Yes.' A rueful grin that made her want to reach up and touch him in sympathy. 'A late one in Emergency last night, but we won. It's a wonder you can't hear my stomach rumbling.'

'No breakfast?'

'No dinner. I really need to stock my fridge with snacks for Mondays when the fast food shops all close early.'

'I guess I could be neighbourly tonight and invite you to dinner, until you get stocked.' Feeling awkward but somehow driven to say it, Nadia added, 'Home-cooked spaghetti bolognese on Tuesday nights. There's always enough left over for an extra person.'

'Can I say yes before you change your mind?'

She smiled at that. 'We eat around six.' Waved him off. 'Katie will probably talk your ear off.'

'Katie has wonderful conversations,' he said and went on his way.

She watched him go straight to the room with the closed door and she knew he'd be pleased at how much little Joseph had improved. Everyone was talking about it this morning.

The day passed swiftly without her seeing Henry again and she cleared her desk and went to pick up Katie.

Afterwards, she and Katie went up to watch the furniture removal people empty the upstairs apartment to take to the new house. Katie had been tasked to help keep Kai amused and out of the way.

'Is Dr Henry moving in soon?' Katie asked as she and Kai built blocks on the kitchen floor. Nadia sighed. Third time she'd heard that question.

Bella cocked her ear at the words and her lips lifted but she spoke to Katie. 'As soon as the cleaners Uncle Simon organised have made it all shiny.'

Nadia heard her sister's wry tone. She knew Bella hadn't been happy with that.

'You should have heard him,' Bella said. Her sister needed a rant, Nadia thought fondly. Hormones and pregnancy—gotta love them all.

Bella lowered her tone to a deep voice that came out very similar to her husband's baritone. 'You can't go cleaning around a pregnant belly.'

Nadia laughed.

Bella went on, 'Which is just ridiculous because I'm as strong as a horse. And pregnancy and birth is a normal thing for women.' She threw up a hand. 'Some women work in the fields until they deliver and then they go on working in the fields with the baby in a sling.'

'Not around here,' said Nadia, laughing. 'In fact, not anywhere in Australia, I think.'

But she did feel secretly glad, after her own eventful pregnancy, that her usually easy-going brother-in-law had put his foot down. Nadia needed everything to go perfectly for her sister after her own disaster. 'You don't want to go into labour exhausted from *silly*—' she used her sister's word '—cleaning that you didn't need to do.'

'Hmm,' said Bella, because there really was no argument to that, and they both watched the last armchair being lifted out of the door. Suddenly, it was all gone. The apartment was empty.

They looked around. Bella said slowly, 'I had so many lovely times here and I will miss the view.'

'But you're more excited about the new house,' said Nadia.

Bella flashed her a big smile. 'Absolutely. I cannot wait to have all the furniture in and sorted.'

Nadia raised her brows but didn't comment that apparently her sister would miss the view but not the relatives she was moving away from.

Bella was quick. 'Oh. That was tactless of me.' She hugged Nadia. 'I will miss you, sis.' She looked down at her niece. 'And of course I'll miss you, Miss Katie. It's been so wonderful being so close and watching you grow up every day.'

Yes, that had been a blessing she should count whenever she missed her sister, Nadia thought.

'We'll come and visit often.'

'And Dr Henry will be here,' said Katie.

Bella laughed. 'He's really made a conquest there, hasn't he?'

'Yes,' said Nadia dryly and Bella tilted her head.

'He hasn't made a conquest of you?'

'Henry is lovely, of course. But he's way too much like Dad. No way I'm going to fall for a man who puts his work first. And the man is a flirt. All the women in the children's ward hang on his every utterance and are offering to follow him home.'

'A flirt? I don't think that's true,' Bella said mildly. 'The flirt thing. Do you think he wants women to follow him home?'

Suddenly, Nadia felt just a little cross with her sister for poking her nose in.

'I don't have any idea what Henry Oliver wants.' And for some reason she didn't mention she'd invited him for pot luck.

'And, sadly, you speak the truth,' said her sister cryptically. 'But I'm off home to make sure these fellows put all the things in the right place. The cleaners will be in tonight.'

'Tonight? Is Henry in that much of a hurry to move in?'

'I imagine so. He's living in a hotel and goodness knows what he's eating. Wouldn't you be?'

And now would be a good time to mention that he was coming for a meal at her apartment tonight. But she didn't. 'Hmm. I suppose so.'

Henry arrived promptly at six p.m. Katie opened the door and gave that little jump up and down she did when she was excited. 'Mummy, it's Dr Henry!'

Nadia, stirring the mince, lifted one hand from the kitchen nook. Seemed he had another fan girl. 'Hello again, Henry. Ask him in, Katie. He's coming for dinner tonight.'

Katie gave another bunny hop. 'Because he's living in a lotel?'

'Hotel,' Nadia corrected with resignation. Big ears.

Henry's amused gaze met hers from the door with a quirk of his brow and she said, 'We watched Bella's removalists upstairs this afternoon and she mentioned you would be moving into the top floor as quickly as possible.' She tilted her head at her daughter. 'Some people don't miss anything.'

Henry laughed, stepped in and closed the door behind him. 'Mummy invited me to have spaghetti bolognese with you tonight, Katie. I don't have a kitchen. Yet.'

'You'll get Auntie Bella's kitchen soon.'

He smiled. 'I will.' Nadia watched him glance around. 'You have a lovely unit, Nadia.'

She warmed at his praise. Yes, she'd tried hard to make it a happy and comfortable home for Katie.

'I always feel like the garden's coming into the house, with the windows and the courtyard. We catch lovely sun in the mornings.'

It was a little awkward. But what did she expect? It had been years since they'd known each other. And there hadn't been that much private conversation during Bella's party.

He was in her home.

'Sit down. Would you like a drink? I have a can of beer left over from when Simon was here a few months ago. I don't know if they go out of date?'

He shook his head, amused. 'No, thanks. I had coffee with a worried dad not long ago.' He smiled and lowered his big body into her couch. He looked good there and she turned towards the kitchen, blocking the picture, in case he read something on her face.

'Then I'll dish up.'

As they ate, Katie carried much of the conversation and, to her surprise, Nadia found Henry's presence unexpectedly restful.

They talked about her photography business a little. He conversed easily with Katie and complimented Nadia's cooking. His obvious enjoyment felt somehow satisfying and she realised she'd missed that feeling of appreciation from a man when she cooked a meal.

A sudden bitter memory of a special meal she and Bella had slaved over for their father's birthday came back to her. He hadn't turned up and later he'd brushed it off, saying he'd already eaten.

Bella had been philosophical but Nadia had cried in her room afterwards. Henry wasn't her father but she wouldn't be getting used to another consultant at her table.

Henry's phone rang not long after they finished and he excused himself, apologised for not helping with the washing-up and left. Nadia felt vindicated by her earlier reservations.

Wednesday she and Katie spent with Bella, helping her open boxes and stack cupboards. With Bella on maternity leave, the move had been good timing to have it done and dusted before the baby arrived.

Thursday had become Nadia's favourite day. Thursday, she enjoyed a full day of photography, shooting scenery, promoting her website and taking or editing portraits for families, and she had a portfolio order to drop off this afternoon.

Katie went to childcare, which she didn't mind on Thursdays as her special friend, Lily, went that day as well.

This morning had been particularly productive, though she hadn't got around to breakfast and suddenly her tummy rumbled at the same time as the phone rang.

She didn't recognise the number. That was the problem with the business number being the same as her private one. She had to answer phone calls even if she didn't know who was on the other end of the line.

'Nadia Hargraves, Hargraves Photography.'

'Nadia, it's Henry.' Deep voice, instant picture—her heartrate did not just leap.

FIONA MCARTHUR   55

Her hand lifted to her chest and then fear
shoved everything else aside. Her throat was suddenly tight. 'Is Katie okay?'

'I thought she went to childcare on Thursdays?'
Henry questioned.

'Yes.' Of course. Childcare would have rung
her. 'She is. Yes.' She felt like slapping her head.
'Sorry. I just had a little panic attack that the doctor was ringing me.'

'No. Sorry.' A pause, then Henry said almost
gently, 'Last thing I want to do is cause you worry.
Not ringing you as a doctor. Is that okay?'

'Of course.' Now she felt super silly.

But Henry hadn't sounded as if he thought she
was silly.

'You said you have Thursdays at home. I wondered if you felt like taking a break and coming
down to the beach café for a quick bite.'

'Did my brother-in-law give you my number?'
And of course he'd tell Bella that Henry had asked
for it. Nadia frowned.

'No.' There was a pause as if he was thinking
through her question. 'I looked up Hargraves Photography.' She suspected he was smiling because
he did sound amused.

'Okay.' She'd pay that. She forgave Simon for
a deed he didn't do. And she was hungry. And
it was only Henry. Only Henry? Nothing 'only'
about Henry, no matter how she pretended.

'I'm a couple of minutes away from our foyer.

You could come down the lift as soon as you're ready. I'll wait.'

She thought about busy Henry waiting. 'No. You go ahead and get a table. It's always busy at lunchtime.'

'I've already booked a table.'

More amusement in his voice. What was so funny? Had he expected her to leap at the offer? She frowned again. Did he think her predictable?

'Not sure of yourself at all?'

'Not at all. I booked for one and said possibly two.'

And that silenced the internal witch. Enough guessing at Henry's motives since she'd got most of it wrong.

'Thank you, Henry, I'm starving, so that would be nice. A walk outside will do me good.'

CHAPTER SIX

Henry

AND SEEING YOU will do me good, thought Henry, delighted she'd agreed. Though she had been slightly combative, which was a little disquieting. Had he annoyed her?

She hadn't sounded overjoyed. Oh, no. It wasn't him she was coming for. It was because she was starving. She needed to get out for a walk.

Lucky he didn't have an ego when it came to women.

That was okay. He'd asked her today to return the hospitality of Tuesday's dinner and he knew she was home on Thursdays and Katie was at childcare.

His thoughts rambled on, creating a scenario he enjoyed. Maybe a casual lunch here and there, depending on their work commitments. She had to eat and so did he.

He liked the idea that she was hungry and he could meet that need for her. Of course, him paying the bill might be a problem but he wouldn't fight about it today if there was a struggle.

Maybe a future dinner date with Simon and Bella, with Nadia and Katie travelling in his car. Simon had mentioned that he and Bella had bought a new child restraint seat for Kai with the new baby coming and hadn't got around to throwing the old one out yet. He could ask for it to keep in his garage if needed for Katie.

Henry was feeling pretty happy today, for some reason.

Nadia swept out of the door of the units just as he reached their steps. Dressed in a knee-length skirt and blue sandals, the cream blouse glued itself to her svelte figure and made her tan glorious. In fact, all of her looked glorious. And then she smiled at him.

There, that was it. That was what he needed in his life.

'Hello, Henry—this is a nice idea.' She smiled sunnily at him. 'But don't think you're going to make a habit of it.'

He blinked, still slightly dazzled. 'Why's that?'

She raised her brows. 'Thursdays are mine.'

Henry thought about that. 'I'm pleased you could come, then. I understand work commitments.' That he did.

'Yes, you would.' Her tone was dry.

No idea what that was about, but he let it go.

'It's a beautiful day,' he said as they began to

walk towards the café. 'I'll be finishing late this evening, so I thought I'd better have a decent lunch in case I don't get dinner.'

She turned her head his way and for a moment he thought he'd said something wrong.

But then she smiled brightly at him. 'Seems to happen often. Working late. Not getting dinner.'

He shrugged. 'Often enough. It's easy to do in a hospital.'

'Lots of after hours, then?' Something in her voice made him cautious.

'I've only been on the ward four days. It's a lot quieter than London.'

She stopped and turned to him, still smiling brightly. 'So, just clarifying, you're one of those doctors who is always there for his patients. Whenever they need him.'

He frowned. 'I hope so. Not much use being someone's doctor if you're not there when needed.' He'd worked darned hard to get where he was and yes, he was a dedicated doctor.

She nodded as if something had been confirmed but they'd arrived at the café and he wondered where that conversation had been going.

He considered his answers. Nothing he would change. But the thoughtful expression on her face said he'd confirmed something for her she'd had a preconceived idea about. It was curious…disquieting. But they'd arrived.

The coffee shop sat perched above Rainbow

Bay, with high stools and tall benches under red umbrellas all facing the waves. Jars of pretty purple-blue knives and forks sat in the middle of the tables. Henry loved the beachy feel to it after London.

The proprietor, a young woman with a dozen piercings, her hair shaved so close to her head it would prickle, grinned at him. 'Henry, your table's over here.' She smiled at Nadia. 'Hello, Nadia. How's Katie?'

'Happy and healthy, thanks, Lulu. And the twins?'

'Full of mischief.' She patted her pocket and pulled out a pen and notebook. 'Want to look at the menu or do you both know what you want and ready to order?' Lulu was used to medical staff in a hurry.

Nadia said, 'I'm ready, thanks, Lulu. I think Henry needs to get back to work and I do too.' She turned her face towards him. 'Is that okay?'

Henry nodded. 'Sure.' Maybe Thursday lunch wasn't going to be the thing.

Nadia said, 'I'll get the smashed avocados and eggs, thanks, Lulu, and a rainbow juice, please.'

'You know your sister orders the same thing when she comes?'

Nadia smiled. 'You do it so well we can't resist.'

Lulu smiled and then lifted her brows at him. Henry allowed his slight tension to slip away. 'And you, Henry?'

Order. Right. Stop thinking disappointed thoughts about his lunch companion's lack of enthusiasm.

'The full all-day breakfast, thanks, Lulu, and a large cappuccino, please.'

'On the way,' she said and winked so of course he winked back.

Nadia sat back in her chair. 'You've only been back in the area a week and already you're Lulu's new fave person?'

He smiled after the waitress slash proprietor. 'She's a gem. Remembered me from when I was here before and welcomed me back like a long-lost friend.'

That bright smile again. 'I can see the ladies do like you.'

He sat back in his own chair and sifted through the messages that were mixed and perturbing. Resisted the urge to say, *I'm sure the men like you too.* Because Nadia was hot.

Instead, he turned his head and allowed his eyes to roam over the bay, before tilting her way and saying calmly, 'I love sitting here. I thought of this exact spot in London when it was sleeting outside. I could see the waves in my mind and the red umbrellas.' He blew out a breath, more settled in himself just remembering that.

Then he shrugged and said very quietly, 'A couple of times I thought of you sitting with me here, when I was in London.'

CHAPTER SEVEN

Nadia

OH. HE DIDN'T just say that. Nadia felt her cheeks heat, mortified. She had no idea why she was in such a foul mood. And taking it out on poor Henry, who didn't do anything wrong except ask her for a friendly lunch.

Still, that tiny picture he'd just painted, so unexpectedly, had derailed her determined hunt to find reasons she shouldn't want to be out for lunch with him. Which was her problem, not Henry's.

This nice man had invited her in the middle of his busy day because he might not have a meal tonight and had asked her to join him.

Here she was whining about a waitress smiling at him when they all knew and loved Lulu, who smiled at everyone. What was wrong with her?

Yes, he spent a lot of time at the hospital, but that wasn't her problem. The fact that he was a caring doctor was a good thing. It didn't mean he was like her father, and while she had to admit it would be a problem for whoever he spent his life with, that too was not her problem.

Because she wouldn't be looking for a part-time husband and a part-time father for Katie. Still, she was jumping way out of line and that thought, and the consequences, were not for today. Or ever.

His last words, though, had whipped the wind from her black sails and stopped her destructive path. She brushed his fingers across the table in apology before drawing back.

'I'm sorry, Henry. Seems I'm a little belligerent today. My bad. I'm out of practice lunching with a man. Haven't done it for years. And you copped my nervousness.'

'Really. That's not a bad thing to hear.' He smiled at her. 'I'm very pleased about that for the past. But allow me.' He waggled his brows. 'I'd be very happy to help you get back into training. Get rid of those nerves for you. Maybe on Thursdays?'

He was teasing. She knew because his brown eyes were twinkling at her and she could see the cute crinkles. Despite herself, she smiled back.

'I'm very protective of my world.'

He nodded solemnly. 'Yes, you told me.'

'And I'm very protective of Katie.' Her voice dropped. 'She's already asked me why she doesn't have a daddy like the other kids at school.' Another huge worry.

'Tricky,' he said, and she could see she had his full attention.

She nodded. 'So I've avoided the idea of her attaching herself to someone who's not around. Or someone who will leave.' She shrugged. 'Hence, I avoid the complications that going out with a man could cause.' But maybe that didn't count with Henry since he was a part of the family and social crowd they circulated with.

She felt her eyes widen as sudden insight penetrated. 'Good grief. It's not just for Katie. I'm scared for me.'

She heard the words. Hadn't meant it to come out. But knew it to be true. She put her hand on her throat.

'That's not so surprising,' he said gently. 'As a widow, your world would have been upended, adrift while grieving. Now you have your world stable. You told me. You want to keep control.'

He did understand, but if she was honest with herself that wasn't the whole problem. She just wondered if he needed to hear the rest of the reasons. And since she didn't want to encourage him—really, she didn't—she guessed he did deserve it.

'Losing someone I loved is a part of it—the death of a spouse does change everything. But there's more to it than that.'

Henry's gaze held hers and he leaned forward,

full attention on her. Softly, he said, 'Can you tell me the *more*?'

How did she explain? She sighed. Henry had been open and honest with her. Could she be the same?

She sat up and straightened her shoulders. 'My husband was a very handsome man. I loved him.' She looked down at the pretty knife and fork she'd put in front of her as she waited for the meal. 'But all women loved him.' She added dryly, 'And... he loved women.'

'Okay,' said Henry, letting her know again she had his full attention.

She went on, 'I don't believe he was unfaithful, but I felt I faded into the background when other women surrounded him. Maybe I was just young and insecure.'

There was silence, not uncomfortable, more of a moment for her to catch her breath after saying things she hadn't said before. Had never allowed herself to think. She appreciated the minute to let it settle.

He touched her hand briefly. Just a quick connection like she'd made and then gone.

'I'm sorry. That must have been hard. But I think he was a fool.' He shook his head, still with that warmth making his brown eyes look very dark and a little too mesmeric. 'He had you. You're amazing. What more could he want?'

She felt her cheeks heat. 'Good grief, Henry. Extravagant compliments today.'

He spread his hands and slid them on the table as if feeling the grain of the wood, a crooked smile on his face. The silence lasted a little while again, not awkward, just both of them…thinking.

She broke it, saying, 'And my husband loved fast cars. He spent almost all of my savings on a stupid car that killed him.' She looked up at him. Narrowed her eyes. 'What type of car do you drive, Henry?'

He laughed. A deep rumbling roll of delight that made her skin prickle and her belly warm. Good grief, that was a sexy laugh. Half the women in the restaurant looked up and smiled.

She watched him force his face into serious lines. 'My car? Oh… It's a Volvo.'

She felt her face pull into a smile, her shoulders sagged as tension left and amusement replaced it. Her turn to laugh.

'You do *not* own a Volvo.'

He smiled at her. 'No. But if it's a deal-breaker for lunches I could buy one.' He was teasing.

'Noted. So you're rich enough to afford a penthouse and a Volvo. And you're a funny man.'

His face looked suddenly serious. 'I'm more than that. Way more. But that's for another day.'

She raised her brows. 'There's another day?'

'Of course.' He rubbed his hands together. 'You've got lots of lunch practice to get in.'

'Spare me,' she said.

'I will. But how about today we just have lunch? Enjoy this beautiful place. With excellent company. Without worrying about the fears and the future.'

She felt her shoulders drop, her facial muscles ease. Even her fingers relaxed.

'Thank you, Henry. I can do that.'

So they did. Until the child at the next table began to choke.

Henry was up and out of his seat, lifting the wheezing, purple-faced toddler out of his high-chair and into his lap while he slipped into a chair at the mother's table. 'Do you mind? I'm a doctor,' she heard him say, and he leant the toddler forward and tapped his open hand firmly between the child's shoulder blades.

Nadia followed—she'd done her emergency first aid certificate, she wouldn't be as useful as her sister Bella or a doctor, but Henry nodded approval. 'Nadia. Great. Can you check his mouth after every tap, and clear it if something dislodges?'

She nodded and crouched down in front of the child as Henry firmly tapped his back. Once. Twice. Three times. The horrible purple of the child's face had deepened, and the mother clutched her throat in panicked terror.

Suddenly, a piece of fruit flew into Nadia's

hand and she whipped it away as the little boy sucked in a gasping breath and wailed.

Henry sat him up and rubbed his back as his breathing settled, despite the cries of distress and fright.

Once Henry was sure the boy would recover he smiled reassuringly at the mother and handed the little boy back.

Lulu appeared beside them and offered a packet of baby wipes to Nadia as she stood up, and one to the mother.

'Oh, good grief, that was frightening. Thank you, Dr Oliver,' Lulu said, making sure everyone heard that Henry was a doctor.

Nadia felt her heart thumping in her chest as her own fear settled. The other patrons sighed in relief and clapped.

They were the centre of attention of smiling fans and she wanted to hide.

They finished their lunch more quickly than they'd previously intended and Henry left her to return to work.

Nadia found herself looking out through the garden window of her unit and staring at the frangipanis more than she should.

He'd thought about her in London.

At least that was what he'd said. A couple of times. Her?

Then it was most likely true, the sensible part

of her brain said. Henry had always been honest. Even when there'd been tough news to share in the NICU he hadn't tried to avoid it.

People trusted him with their unwell kids. Huge trust. The woman today had trusted him to save her child. And the children's ward already adored him.

She thought about his sincerity as he'd held her gaze and said those startling words. He'd thought of her. Thought of her in London. But only a couple of times.

Henry had moral fibre. She struggled with the thought because she didn't want to label Alex, her husband, a dead man, as lacking, but yes, really, she'd loved a man who hadn't existed. Her husband had lacked maturity, responsibility and principle and she'd grown a strong wall around her heart after he'd died. She wasn't likely to fall into that silliness again.

Henry was different, but she still wasn't willing to let him in. Henry was reliable and honourable and honest, which for her was one of the most important qualities in a man. And apparently Henry liked her.

She thought of the drama of the café and the fact that Henry would always be the doctor who rushed in to save. Like her dad. That was a good thing, a great thing. Did that make her a bad person because she didn't want any of it?

* * *

At two p.m. she packed the new portfolio into a protective folder and took her car out of the underground garage to drive to her client's house. She didn't drive all the time, except for her photography business and picking up Katie from the preschool and shopping days—otherwise, everything else, including work, was within a short stroll. Though now they'd have to drive to Bella's new house.

The road seemed busy, and she decided she'd ask Gran if she wanted to come with her out to Bella's when she picked Katie up from daycare. Gran didn't like driving on busy days.

Most of all, both Gran and her sister were sensible women who would listen to her ridiculous anxiety over going to lunch with the first man since becoming a widow.

Nadia's grandmother, Catherine Goodwin Hargraves, had been an adventurer in her youth. She'd slowed down now, especially after a nasty hit-and-run accident five years ago that had left her unconscious for weeks, but now her green eyes, so like her great-granddaughter's, although faded slightly, were clear and shrewd.

If it hadn't been for Gran, Nadia and Bella wouldn't have had anything like a normal childhood. They would have spent their holidays locked in the house with part-time nannies, waiting for a crumb of attention from their workaholic father, but instead they had Gran, always smiling and suggesting adventures perfect for children.

When they were teenagers, Gran had moved to Rainbow Bay to look after an ailing sister who had since passed away, and the girls had started flying up from Sydney for occasional weekends when they were older.

For Nadia, living in the same block of units with Gran and Bella had been an incredible support after she'd brought Katie home from hospital. And the inclusive family she and Katie had been surrounded with still felt priceless.

'Have you been out with anyone yet?' said Gran, forthright as usual as soon as she was settled.

Bella thought how typical that statement was as a conversation starter. She'd been hearing it a lot for the last few months. To give her grandmother some leeway, Nadia knew the accident had shaken Catherine's world view of being here for many years to come. She wanted Nadia settled before she died. Hopefully married with more children.

Nadia concentrated on navigating the busy streets to Bella's new house. Katie was in her booster seat in the back, immersed in a singalong on her tablet which was connected to the rear of the passenger seat, and hopefully would miss the opportunity to hear this and repeat it at the most awkward moment.

'Well, I went to an impromptu lunch with Henry Oliver today. Does that count?' She didn't mention the neighbourly dinner.

'Did you?' Her grandmother straightened in her seat. 'I like Henry. A caring man, I feel.' Nadia could sense the searching look coming her way, but she refused to intercept it. 'And how was lunch?'

Nadia kept her expression serene. She badly wanted to say, *Sometimes awkward, sometimes wonderful*, but didn't.

'Fine, until a child choked and Henry saved the day.'

'Good grief, how horrible. What happened?'

'A piece of apple happened. Then Henry was up, boy on his lap bent forward and striking the little chap on the back. The apple dislodged.' She thought of that happening to Katie and shuddered. At least she'd been reminded to know instantly what to do. 'I'm glad he was there.'

'I'm sure the mother of the child was as well. How horrid for everyone.'

'Yes. All very dramatic and it sort of ruined the lunch.'

'I imagine so.' She felt her grandmother's gaze on her. 'And before the drama? How was lunch before that?'

'Pleasant.' Nadia flicked a quick glance to see the response.

'Pleasant.' Catherine moved her mouth as if the word was distasteful.

Nadia turned back to the road and grinned.

'I'm so pleased,' Catherine said dryly. 'I would have preferred delightful, exciting, great fun. But I'll take pleasant. At least he asked you.'

'What makes you think I didn't ask him?'

'My own lamentable lack of imagination,' her grandmother said dryly.

True, but not very complimentary.

'Are you saying I wouldn't have asked Henry out myself?'

'Yes.'

Well, she had asked him to dinner. So there. But Nadia only laughed.

'Okay, he rang me on his way walking past and said he was going for lunch. He had a big afternoon at work coming up and needed a decent meal.'

'Poor man.' Catherine tsked. 'He needs a wife.'

Not this little black duck, Nadia thought, so she ignored that.

'I was hungry, so I said yes.'

'Good, because he's a very *pleasant* young man.' Copying Nadia's description. Silence built between them. The faint strains of a child's song drifted from the back.

Nadia remembered Henry's words and almost blurted, *He says he's more than that*, but she didn't.

Finally, she said very quietly, 'We went to the beach café. Glorious weather. All done within an hour, including the excitement. And I may have behaved badly at the start.'

Catherine drew in a surprised breath. 'Did you? Strange. You never behave badly.'

'Well, only initially. And thank you for that vote of confidence. But I was extremely snarky with Henry.'

'Really?' She could feel her gran's scrutiny. 'What about? And why?'

'Stupid things. Women fawning over him. His workload. My world I was protecting.'

'Good grief.' Gran snorted. 'Did he enjoy the fireworks?'

'He seemed fine. I said I was out of practice with men.'

Gran turned in her seat to look at her. 'You are. Very.' She smiled. 'And what did he say?'

'Henry said he'd help me get back into training.'

Gran laughed. 'I do like this boy. Though I'm not sure a bare hour for lunch constitutes going out, but it's a start.'

'Thank you. But I'm not looking for a man. Yet.'

'I see. So when? It's more five years, dear.'

'Gently, gently, Gran.'

'Yes, dear,' murmured Catherine.

CHAPTER EIGHT

Henry

HENRY'S AFTERNOON PROVED too busy, working with the excellent team at the children's ward, to be able to dwell on his lunch with Nadia. He smiled and made decisions and concentrated on each diagnosis.

Yet every time he had a free moment Nadia's face seemed always there at the back of his mind, and he thought of that word she'd used. Scared.

Well, yes, shocking, but it made sense if she was feeling threatened by the concept of forming a relationship. And it had worked in his favour while he'd been away because she wasn't settled with someone else. But still, he felt sad that such a beautiful woman had those limitations in her life.

As long as she didn't feel threatened by him—or the concept of him intruding into the safety of her world—he could see how a shift in her world view as a single parent would be a valid concern for her.

So, what were her other fears? And why was he so intrigued when Nadia's signals today had been mixed at best?

Judging by the veiled accusations of him being a ladies' man—which was just not true—and something about spending excessive time at the hospital—which couldn't be helped—it was probably linked with her past. He just had to find out what it was.

Her deceased husband was the easy answer. She'd intimated the man had a roving eye at the very least.

He'd actually spent the plane trip home from the UK alternating between wondering if she was still single since the last time he'd asked her brother-in-law, an irregular occurrence, and fantasising about how he would find her if she was.

And the answer to that, after today's revelations, was cautious. He needed to talk to Simon.

When Henry had finished his tasks, he took himself through the hospital to the NICU—Neonatal Intensive Care Unit—which was Simon's domain.

His friend stood conversing with Carla, the unit's nurse manager and a friendly face from the past.

Carla looked up and greeted him with a smile. 'Hello, Henry. Lovely to see you. I heard you were back.'

'Greetings, Carla. Love your new hairstyle.'

'Goodness, London has polished you.' But she patted her hair.

'Ah, I've been trained by a master. My Italian flatmate encouraged me to actually appreciate little things like that.' He remembered Nadia's accusations, grinned at her and held up his hands. 'Not flirting.'

Carla laughed. 'Good to know.'

'The unit looks great.'

She smiled with delight. 'Happy to take the compliment. We have great staff. How are you enjoying the children's ward?'

'Ditto on the great staff.'

'Yes, clever bunch over there,' said Carla. 'And the new refurbishment is great. I'm guessing you've come to talk to Simon, so I'll leave you to your discussion.'

Simon studied him with a slight smile on his face.

Henry put his hands out. 'What?'

'Something for later. And you did come back smooth.'

'Maybe, and maybe it's a problem,' he said. 'I think I need a buddy pep talk.'

Simon smiled. 'Walk me to my car.' He glanced at his watch. 'I'm late for dinner and I try not to be.'

Henry's head went up. 'Is that a big deal?'

'Yes. Because Bella and Nadia's father… You've met the professor?'

'No, I don't think I have.'

'A joy waiting for you, then.' Simon beeped his car open but didn't get in.

Henry stilled as all denominations of coins fell and pushed the right recognition buttons. 'Oh...'

'Right. Solved one of your problems already, have I?'

'Maybe. Thanks.' He patted Simon's arm. 'You should go.'

Simon smiled, went to climb in and then stopped. 'You said maybe coming back "smooth" would be a problem. Why?'

Henry sighed. 'I went to lunch with Nadia today.'

'Fast work.' Simon grinned. 'Not surprised, but I'm impressed.'

'Impromptu. Anyway, do you know anything about her ex-husband?'

Simon's grin faded. 'A bit. But that's Nadia's business. Ask her.'

'I will. But not soon. I'm going slow.' In fact, he wasn't even sure he had the qualities Nadia wanted in a man—apparently, he was like her father.

Looking thoughtful, Simon considered that. 'Very wise. Come around on the weekend. See the new house. Borrow the car seat.' He grinned. 'If you think it's safe to pull it out this early.'

'Might not be a good idea just yet.' Henry thought about the belligerent Nadia he'd first met outside the units, not presuming anything, and he expected to be busy at work this weekend as his registrar was away on a course. 'But thanks.'

CHAPTER NINE

Nadia

NADIA AND CATHERINE arrived at Bella's new house at Bilinga and were greeted by the new housekeeper, Mrs Tierney, a plump, perpetually smiling woman with pepper and salt hair who ushered them in with undisguised delight.

The two-storey house sat barely four kilometres from the hospital and across the road from the grassy Bilinga Beach, one of the quietest beaches on the Gold Coast, with sand and sea beyond. The yard had a tall surrounding fence with electronic gates and was set on a double block with a gorgeous outdoor entertainment area.

The well-fenced pool came with a children's slide and spa for the adults. The house itself held six bedrooms and four bathrooms. Nadia agreed with Bella's husband that her sister needed a housekeeper and possibly a gardener.

If Bella hadn't been pregnant and on maternity leave she might have complained more strenuously about the idea of needing help twice a week, but for the moment she'd adapted to the idea. And struck gold.

Nadia knew Mrs Tierney came in on Tuesdays and Thursdays and Mr T accompanied his wife and managed the gardens. Already, Kai had taken a shine to Mr T and the gruff Irishman, who only slightly resembled a garden gnome because of his rounded low stature and beard, allowed the little boy to watch him as he pruned and tended the flowerbeds.

Not long after Nadia and her grandmother followed Mrs T through the house, Katie took herself off after Mr T as well and pelted him with questions.

'Let's have a cup of tea in the sitting room before Mr and Mrs T go home,' said Bella. 'Before the children come back in.'

Gran said, 'Where did you find that delightful couple?'

'So fortunate.' Bella smiled at the memory. 'Simon looked after their daughter's premature baby last year, and we ran into them one day at the shops, both looking very woebegone.

'Mr T asked if we had any gardening he could do as they'd sold their house and moved into a unit.'

'Ah. Yes, I understand that,' said Catherine, who'd always had a green thumb.

Nadia smiled and didn't comment. She kept

fake plants in the house to save the death and destruction she caused to anything with real leaves but the garden on the other side of the low wall that gave her such pleasure was maintained by the units and flourished gloriously.

Bella went on. 'While we were talking, we discovered their daughter and husband had had to move away for work, and the couple missed their grandchild dreadfully. Said their lives felt empty except for the times they performed their duties as traffic wardens for the school near their home. Mornings, they patrol the zebra crossing for the children who cross to school between seven and nine a.m.'

Nadia glanced at Gran, who raised her brows.

Bella waved her hand. 'They're great. She manages me, just by smiling sweetly. Simon's delighted. So yes, I think I work for them rather than the other way round.'

'Well, your house looks like you've lived here for years.' Nadia gazed around in wonder.

'Good,' said Gran. 'I'm pleased. It always amazes me how many women move house when heavily pregnant. Such a lot of work when you've got a busy time coming up.'

Bella smiled. 'Yes, you made your view very clear when we first mentioned we were moving. I thought you'd be happy that I have some help.'

She turned to Nadia. 'But enough about me. Tell me about your world. How's life in the units since I've gone? How's business? Have you seen much of Henry?'

Nadia didn't look at her grandmother. 'Life's good. Photography's doing well. And, ah, yes, I went to lunch with Henry today, as a matter of fact.' Again, no mention of the dinner because then she'd be interrogated by Gran for not mentioning it. She wished she'd never invited him. A small voice inside whispered, *Liar.*

'Did you?' Bella didn't quite clap her hands, but she looked very pleased.

Nadia tried to play it down. 'It was just an impromptu friendly lunch.'

'Sure. Of course it was.' Her sister leaned towards her. 'You know he fancies you, don't you?'

Nadia remembered his comment that he'd thought of her in London, but she wasn't sharing that. Again, not sure why.

'I'm not looking for a man.'

'Keep telling yourself that. One day you will.' Bella sat back as Mrs T put a tray with a teapot and cups in front of them. 'Thank you, dear Mrs T.'

The older woman smiled serenely and left.

Gran murmured, 'No reason two pleasant people can't get together.'

'It was one lunch.' *Spare me, Gran*, thought Nadia. 'It wouldn't work with Henry. You know as well as I do that he works long hours. And probably will for the rest of his working life. He belongs to the hospital.'

Bella raised her brows at that. 'He works with Simon too.'

'Yes. A full load. I don't want to live with someone like Dad again. And I certainly don't want my daughter to have a fragment of a part-time father either.'

Gran interjected, 'Your sister's managed to make it work.'

Nadia sighed. 'Yes, but Simon's an established consultant. He can make his own rules. Henry is just starting out and I understand that he wants to be there for everyone.'

Gran harrumphed but Bella nodded. 'I understand that. And I have to admit it was a sticking point for Simon and me.'

Despite Bella's agreement, there was something determined and older-sisterish in her eyes that portended advice that might prove unpalatable.

Silence, except for the muted sound of tea pouring into cups, hung heavy over the table.

Gran groaned loudly. 'Your father has a lot to answer for. Problems in Bella's relationship. Difficulties with Simon's workload. And now you. I'm sorry for you girls. I'm sorry I didn't do enough to see that Piers' obsession with work didn't damage you.'

They both leaned forward. 'You did so much, Gran. You were amazing,' said Bella.

'Every holiday, most weekends. And always at the end of the phone,' added Nadia.

Catherine didn't look happy. 'Yes, I tried. But you're still scarred by it, aren't you?'

This conversation had turned out way more depressing than Nadia had thought it would. 'No, Gran. It's not just that.'

She looked at her sister. 'I've been married. I know what it's like to fall madly in love with someone and then to come second to something else in their life.' She shrugged. 'After the freedom I've had for the last few years I'm not sure I want to do that again.'

Gran huffed. 'Apples and oranges. Henry is twice the person that man was.'

'You never liked Alex?' Nadia blinked. 'You never said.'

'Not my place. But I'm sorry, dear, no. Didn't trust him as far as I could throw him.' Seeing that Gran was about twenty centimetres shorter than Nadia's husband had been, that wouldn't have been far, and Nadia decided to redirect this uncomfortable conversation.

Besides, she had another good reason.

'Katie's got all of me now.' Nadia held Bella's gaze. 'Think of all the disappointments when Dad didn't come to school events. The awards. Graduations.'

'Simon will be there for our children,' said Bella firmly.

Nadia opened her mouth to dispute that, but her sister held her hand up. 'Katie sharing you is a good thing. Plus, one day Katie will go away and have a life of her own, so you have to make yours. You'll be the person who gave her everything and was left behind.'

Gran huffed again. 'And I have to mention that you have no male friends, so any male role model would be an extra.'

So much for *support*, Nadia thought gloomily as her grandmother sat back, having made her point. All this because of one lunch. And they didn't even know about the dinner. That would teach her to break her own rules.

CHAPTER TEN

Henry

HENRY DIDN'T HAVE time to run into Nadia over the weekend. He'd spent most of Saturday and Sunday in and out of the hospital at all hours, arriving home after midnight.

Devlin, the four-year-old boy he'd spent most of the time with, had remained in Intensive Care but was improving after Henry had treated the correct diagnosis.

His resident had admitted the child with scarlet fever, but the little boy's red, cracked lips and his swollen tongue had raised Henry's suspicions. Even the palms of Devlin's hands and feet had been swollen and red. And peeling.

Henry had seen Kawasaki disease in London and had been quick to instigate the treatment of gamma globulin. Crucially, they needed to prevent heart damage for Devlin, something that could happen if treatment didn't commence promptly.

This morning, Henry felt a quiet satisfaction with Devlin's recovery and lack of new symptoms, and the young boy looked on track to be transferred back to the children's ward today.

On his way to discuss the good news and the boy's admission with Tara Taylor, the idea of seeing Nadia at her desk at the front of the children's ward quickened his step. He hadn't managed to pass either Nadia or her grandmother in their mutual foyer for days.

And there she was. Henry blew out a breath he hadn't realised he'd been holding. His very own daffodil on a busy day, easing the tension in his neck just by seeing her.

Except she wasn't his.

A small red warning light came on in his brain. *Be careful*, it blinked. *Slow down. If Nadia can't feel the way you do, then what are you doing? You don't have time to pursue someone who has reservations.*

She looked up and saw him and that smile she sent him extinguished his little red warning light with a pop of disdain. Ha! She wasn't immune to him.

His mouth curved with pleasure. 'Good morning, Nadia. You are just what I need to see on a Monday morning. You look wonderful.'

'Thank you.' Her smile faded as she studied him. 'Can't say the same for you, Henry. Looks like you've had no sleep. Again.' She lifted her gaze higher. 'Have you been pulling your hair?'

At least she saw him, then. She even noticed his tiredness. Excellent, he thought, if a bit flattening that she thought he looked rough.

'If I bend so you can reach, will you pat my spikes down?'

'No.' The answer was short, but the smile had returned to her sapphire eyes and she shook her head. 'No PDAs here.'

'Happy to go somewhere else?'

She had him. Yep. Something about this woman…

She raised her brows in *This is work* disapproval. But he just knew she was holding back amusement.

To redeem himself he semi-explained. 'One of my patients. A little boy who's been very sick is on the mend. I haven't had the relaxing weekend I expected, but he's recovering now so it's all worth it.'

He watched her brows draw together and remembered her accusation that he lived at the hospital.

'Of course.' She looked away and that movement caught his attention. She nodded, not looking at him, staring at something else. 'It always is.'

'We'll bring him downstairs today.' He didn't know why their mood had flattened, but he wouldn't talk about little Devlin here. He was tired. She was acting oddly. Best strategy might be to exit until his brain started working better. 'Is Tara in?'

'Just back from a department heads meeting. She could be in the staffroom if she's not in her office.'

'Right, thanks.' He nodded and forced himself to leave her and get on with his work.

He didn't get to talk to Nadia again that day, though he dropped by a couple of times because he still felt uneasy but, not finding her at her desk, he shrugged his unease away.

When a surgical consult about a child with a ruptured appendix kept him busy until she'd disappeared home, he didn't have time to think of her again.

On Thursday Henry warned his secretary that he really needed to have a lunch break today. Often, he just worked through if there were appointments that needed urgent consults.

Today, his plan included mooting the idea to Nadia about him driving her and Katie to Simon and Bella's proposed house-warming barbecue on Saturday.

Most of all, he just wanted to sit down with Nadia in a pretty place and spend time with her. And maybe make up for the last drama filled lunch. But he still hadn't called her. She'd been difficult to pin down on Monday and Tuesday, except for that first sighting of her at the beginning of his workday, and he'd thought he'd catch sight of her or Katie before now, out and about.

Nope. That hadn't happened. He found himself hoping it was bad luck and not machinations on her part to avoid him.

He shrugged and pressed her number.

'Hargraves Photography.'

'It's Henry. How are you?'

'Good, thanks, Henry.' A brief pause. 'You?'

'Fine. I'm passing for lunch in a little while and wondered if I could entice you out again. Try for a non-drama-filled lunch. Surely lightning can't strike twice in the same place?' He found himself a little too invested in the answer.

'Well, I haven't eaten.' A pause. Reluctance? 'Thank you. What time are you thinking of going?'

Relief sagged his shoulders. This was ridiculous and he needed to work through her reluctance or drop the whole idea of pursuing Nadia.

'My last patient is at twelve so, all going well, say twelve thirty-five.'

'Same place? You've booked a table?'

'I have. For one, maybe two.' It amused him to remind her about her comment of him being sure of her last time.

'Then that sounds fine. Are you planning on phoning me every Thursday, Henry?' There was wryness in her tone and he felt himself smile though she couldn't see him.

'I'd like to do more than that, but yes, I'll settle for Thursdays at the moment.'

Maybe he shouldn't have said that.

There was a pause and she murmured, 'I see. Then, in that case, I'll choose where we go next Thursday.'

Relief washed through him again. 'Absolutely. Sounds great—we could alternate with choices.'

'There's going to be that many Thursdays?'

'That's the plan. I'll see you outside the units. At twelve thirty-five.'

Ridiculously, his heart felt as light as one of those seagulls flying outside his window. *Careful.*

CHAPTER ELEVEN

Nadia

SO THERE WAS a plan? Nadia thought as she put her phone down, and she couldn't help admitting she might just have missed him the last few days.

As long as she was careful. If Henry was looking for a relationship, she needed to make up her mind if she was interested or too…scared? Scarred? Sensible? She wanted to… But something dark and frightened inside her still wasn't sure what she wanted.

It seemed dishonest not to tell him he might be better spending his time with someone else, unless he wasn't looking long-term. Ooh, a fling? No.

Asking for that wouldn't be awkward much. No!

She shook her head at her idiocy and glanced at the clock. She had an hour before lunch and thirty minutes of work to do before then. Maybe she'd think of something to say.

She really tried to work. But it was hard to concentrate. Thoughts of when she'd seen him on Monday morning and how tired he looked. How she'd avoided him on Tuesday, catching glimpses and forcing herself to go the other way.

Henry had moved in upstairs and there was a little ridiculous pique at not being invited to see what he'd done with the big space. He had her number.

Then there were the thoughts of him going upstairs and grabbing whatever he could from the cupboard to eat after a long day. Going to bed and getting up again to answer calls.

She liked Henry. She really did. Liked him a lot.

But all the markings of someone who just wouldn't be there for her and Katie were bright and clear for anyone with her past experience.

She'd seen how consultants could be sucked into immersion at the hospital…have no other lives…desert their families. Thoughts of all those disappointing moments in her childhood when her dad had not been there resurfaced. But this was Henry, she had to remind herself.

She didn't want that to happen to Henry's family. Or have Henry make it happen to her family. Because no, she didn't want it to happen to her and Katie.

But right now, she needed to get this portfolio

of baby photos completed and get herself to the front door by twelve thirty-five.

She was early. She saw him walking up the street at a brisk pace, on his phone, probably crisis managing long-distance. She'd seen her father with his phone in his hand all her life.

But this tall, handsome man wasn't her father, she reminded herself. Instead, she forgot to think and just watched. She drew in the sight of him, striding, confident, smiling at the world as he talked the whole time. The glints of gold in his brown hair that hung a little bit too long for fashion over his brow. His strong shoulders stretching the button-up shirt, sleeves rolled up, showing powerful arms. Long, confident strides towards her, strides that quickened when he saw her waiting.

Nadia couldn't deny the flutter of excitement and warmth that leapt inside her. Oh, dear. That flutter was a worry.

'Hello, Nadia.' The words were deep and soft, like the smile on his face, and the warmth turned into a hot glow curling like melting toffee spiralling inside her.

Henry leaned forward and kissed her cheek, his mouth warm and firm against her skin.

She hadn't expected that. Her surprise must have shown on her face because he stepped back and said, 'It's always so good to see you.'

'Nice to see you too, Henry.' She resisted the impulse to touch her face where his lips had been. She was seriously out of practice with a man.

Had she always been this awkward?

Had men always been this smooth?

What did other women do? No, she couldn't go there. Henry would have to deal with what Nadia did. 'No dinner for you tonight, again?'

They started walking, their steps easily falling into a rhythm that matched.

His brows went up in mock surprise. 'Are you offering to feed me again?'

She spluttered. 'No!'

'Shame.' He quirked a grin, then turned his expression to mournful and sighed. 'My cupboards are bare and it's takeaway Thursday.'

She refused to feel sorry for him. He'd made his choices.

'Poor you. What you need is a housekeeper now you have a home. To leave you a meal and shop.'

The grin came back. 'Are you looking for a job?'

She spluttered again. 'No!'

He patted her shoulder, his fingers warm and strong against her bare skin. 'I'm joking. I'm fine. I just want lunch.' A brief pause. 'With you.'

There he was again, flirting.

'I'll get Simon onto you. He believes in outsourcing to make time. He'll get you a housekeeper.'

They arrived at the beach café and Lulu waved to a well-positioned table for two. Menus lay on the table beside a bottle of water.

Henry pulled out her chair and, when she was seated, sat down himself and poured two glasses of the water.

'Cheers,' he said as he held his glass up.

'Cheers,' she repeated, and they clinked glasses. She couldn't help smiling. 'I believe this is a wonderful vintage.'

'Oh, I agree,' mused Henry, his expression pulled serious. 'I think it's the tangy quality of the chlorine that makes it particularly palatable.'

She nodded sagely. Took another sip. 'Young. Fresh. A bold little white.'

They laughed. It was so silly, but sitting here with Henry, shaded from the sun by their red umbrella, the ocean in front of them, it was even more delightful than last time.

'You have no idea how much I enjoy hearing you laugh,' Henry said.

'Why, thank you, kind sir.' Despite the flippant reply, Nadia remembered that moment last week when he'd thrown back his head and done the same. 'I enjoy your laugh too.' And all the women in the restaurant had smiled, drawn to him. There was that. Her mood flattened a little.

He leaned forward. 'Do you know I've fancied you from the first moment I saw you in that wheelchair, coming to visit Katie in the NICU?'

He said the most astonishing things. She thought back to that hazy time. 'You mean sick, wild-haired, in a hospital gown?'

His expression softened and he shook his head minutely. 'Your hair like gold, you were pale, beautiful, and you had a blue dressing gown,' he corrected her. 'But I found out you were newly widowed and had a prem baby demanding all of your attention. And you were my patient's mother.'

She didn't know what to answer to that. Where to look. This was unexpectedly frank of him.

She managed, 'I must admit it's all a blur back there.'

His gaze held hers, gentle but sincere. 'The time wasn't right for me to intrude. I knew you needed your family around you, I needed to advance my career and, like the song, London was calling.'

'I'm sure you had a wow of a time in London,' Nadia replied, trying to lighten the mood.

His warm gaze didn't leave hers. 'Nobody in London matched up to you.'

She sucked in a breath. 'Stop flattering me.'

Heavy praise she didn't quite believe. And she'd had no idea he fancied her back then. Though the thought did strange things to her squirmy stomach. Things she told herself she didn't want to think about.

He tutted. 'Truth, not flattery. I told you I only went out with the girlfriends of my flatmate's girlfriend.' He shook his head sadly. 'Poor Marco was always devastated I wouldn't go on a second date with any of them.'

Striving for composure, she said, hopefully in a disbelieving tone, 'I'm sure your work took up most of your time.' But she was thinking, *No second dates at all?*

He shrugged. 'Work. Of course. That's why I was there. But no women I remember like I remembered you.' The words were soft but sincere and slid past her guard like a silver arrow.

Oh, my. Her sister's words came back to her. *'One day Katie will go away and make a life of her own, so you have to make yours.'* Was she being stupid to push a man like Henry away before seeing what they could have together, too scared to even try?

Thankfully, Lulu arrived with her notebook and pencil, and Nadia looked up, so relieved she offered a huge smile. Lulu looked tired.

'Hey, Lulu, how are the boys?'

'Jake is home from school with a sore throat and terrible aches and pains. Haven't had much sleep. My mother's minding him.'

'I'm sorry.' She hated when Katie was sick, though it didn't happen often. 'Kids get sick fast, don't they. Hope they get better even faster. Fingers crossed that's soon.'

Henry nodded. 'Most recover quickly. But if the boys are not any better tomorrow, bring them into

Emergency, Lulu. I'll get my resident to phone me when they come in and I'll check them out for you.'

'Thank you.' A wan smile for Henry. 'I will.'

Henry frowned at the worry clear on Lulu's face. 'If you're concerned you can bring them earlier. You know that, right?'

'I will. Thanks, Henry.' She lifted the notebook. 'What can I get you two?'

Henry looked at Nadia to order first and she stared at her menu. Her brain still swirled from his comments and her stomach still twirled in a dance she didn't seem to be able to stop. Menu. Right. She needed something heavy to sit on her belly and make it stay still.

'I'll go for a chicken burger, please, Lulu. And a skim latte. Thanks.'

'Got it. Henry?'

'That sounds good. Same, except I have a full cappuccino in a mug, thanks.'

She hurried off when someone waved at her.

'Poor Lulu. She looks stressed.'

'She does.' Henry watched her walk away. 'I hope the boys feel better soon. She seems very concerned. I'll talk to her again before we leave.'

Above and beyond.

'That's very nice of you, Henry.'

'Not really. But I promised you lunch.' He smiled at her. 'Back to our conversation. The one I started when we arrived here, and when we spoke on the phone.'

She picked up her water and sipped because suddenly her mouth felt dry. 'Oh?' was all she could manage, still hiding behind her glass.

He reached across and gently pulled her hand down so he could see her face. 'I want to see you more than just lunch on Thursdays, Nadia. I'd like to take you to dinner. Maybe a trip with you and Katie in my car. Even if we just go to see Bella and Simon to start.' He was watching her with too much focus.

He'd included Katie and her sister in his plans. He really did have plans. 'Um… What do you want me to say?'

He gave a short laugh but there wasn't much humour in it, which seemed out of character. 'I'd like you to say what you think and feel about that.'

Well, that dropped the conversation on her side of the table. All the things she should say warred with wanting to say, *Yes, I'd like that, Henry.* Because who wouldn't enjoy his company? But in fact she didn't want to fall for Henry, which she knew could be very, very easy to do. She had promised herself Katie would not have the life her dad had given her and Bella.

Instead, she said, 'Well, of course that's very pleasant…' She had a sudden thought of her grandmother grimacing at the word. 'Really lovely,' she amended. Though that wasn't much

better. 'Thank you,' she hastily added on. 'But…'
Nadia drew a breath and squared her shoulders
'… I'm worried about you, Henry. I'm very happy
to become friends. But I'm not planning on a relationship. And from some of the things you've
said, I'm guessing you're coming from a different place. I've told you I'm happy with my own
status quo.'

He watched her thoughtfully, the silence a little more strained this time. Finally, he said, 'And
that leaves me where?'

Fair enough.

'So as long as you're aware of my reluctance to
commit, I'm sure I'd enjoy going out with you.'

He sat back. 'Do you find me attractive at all?'

She raised her brows. Almost snorted. 'You're
joking, right?' Had to laugh. Pointed her finger
at the centre of his awesome chest. 'Look at you.
You're a hunk, Henry. Gorgeous. It's not that.'

He smiled, his cheeks a little pink at her comments, which made her smile again.

'More information than I expected,' he said.
'Thank you. So do you mean by not being in a
relationship that you'd be free to date other men?'

Her eyes went wide. 'Good grief, no, I wouldn't
do that.' She laughed. 'Haven't dated in the last
five years, so not that.' *Apart from lunch with you*,
but she didn't say that. 'Except for social events
with Bella and Simon, I don't get to dress up,
go out at all. You know? Have fun. With adults.

You're offering me that and I'd be crazy not to say that sounds like fabulous fun.'

'Better. Fabulous fun is good.' He tilted his head. 'So, you're saying if I'm willing to risk my heart you're happy to spend time with me? With Katie, on jaunts around town.'

She thought about that.

'Yes.' But there was some reluctance and she suspected he didn't miss it.

He didn't comment on that. 'Good. How about I take you and Katie to Simon and Bella's barbecue on Saturday, instead of us taking two cars?'

She blinked. That had come out of left field. He'd had that ready. 'I was going to take Gran.'

'We can include your grandmother as well. Lots of room in my Volvo.'

She laughed. 'Bought one this week, did you?'

'No, but there's room in my other car.'

Still smiling, she nodded. That actually sounded good, she decided.

'Lovely. Thank you. I might even be able to enjoy a glass of wine, which I can't if I'm driving.'

'Excellent. I'll pick you and your little family up at your door on Saturday at eleven.'

The word manoeuvre came to mind. Had Henry just manoeuvred her? With perfect timing, their meal and drinks arrived in a rushed slither at that moment.

'Sorry,' Lulu said and turned away.

'Lulu.' He caught her sleeve and she spun towards him. Her normally mobile face looked strained and frightened.

'What's happening?'

'Oh, Henry… Jake went to lie down after lunch. I thought he was just tired. But he woke up with a stiff neck and now he has a raging temperature and my mum said he's taken a turn for the worse. I have to go upstairs.' Lulu lived above the shop.

Henry stood without hesitation, though he did glance at Nadia briefly in apology. 'I'll come with you, Lulu.' He touched Lulu's arm.

Nadia blinked. But another look at Lulu's stricken face and she was up too. 'I'll come as well. Maybe I can help.'

'What about your lunch?' Lulu looked torn.

Nadia brushed that away. 'I'll ask them to make it takeaway and then follow you both upstairs.'

In the surprisingly spacious flat above the café Henry took one look at Jake and said to Nadia, 'Please call an ambulance.'

She could do that. At least she could be useful.

To Lulu he said, 'Jake needs to be in the hospital. I'll stay until the ambulance arrives and then I'll meet you in Emergency.' Lulu sank onto a chair and covered her face but she was nodding.

When the paramedics came more quickly than expected, Nadia shooed Lulu away with Jake. 'I'll bring your overnight bag.' Henry sent her a grateful look and left at a brisk walk when they did.

She stayed with Lulu's mother and his frightened twin brother, Jackson, until the necessities were packed, phone chargers and a change of clothes and toiletries for Jake and Lulu. This was Henry's medical world, not hers.

But ten minutes later, after picking up their boxed lunches, Nadia carried the small overnight backpack past her own unit and on to the hospital for Lulu. As she walked, she mused on the fact that, yes, here was another interruption to spending time with Henry. But what was happening to Lulu as another single mum, and a friend of sorts, made Nadia's heart thump in fear.

The fact that Henry proved a hopeless lunch companion was a moot point. Thank God for him being there for Jake.

CHAPTER TWELVE

Henry

ONCE HE ARRIVED in Emergency, Henry saw his registrar had already found Lulu and the paramedics. Jake was being pushed into a cubicle.

When the ambulance personnel left, the petite registrar lifted her head and spoke concisely. 'I've taken bloods, sir, and because of his stiff neck asked the nurses to set up for a lumbar puncture.'

It was so good to see Amelia more confident as each week passed. He'd kept telling her she was brilliant and to use her instincts.

Henry nodded. 'I will be doing that. And your examination?'

'Jake's drowsy, slightly confused to which day it is, and sensitivity to light is noted as well as the stiff neck.'

'No vomiting?'

'No.'

'What about a rash?'

'Not that I saw, but they're changing him now into a gown so visibility will be better.'

'Okay, let's go see him.' He touched the distraught mum's arm. 'Come on, Lulu, you're with us.'

Henry's second impression confirmed that Jake looked very unwell. The nine-year-old was usually robust and noisy. The fast-breathing, pale and limp child in front of Henry made his own heart-rate spike.

'What are his observations?'

Amelia repeated them instantly. 'Temperature's thirty-nine. Pulse one-forty. Blood pressure eighty on fifty.'

All signs of galloping infection.

'How long ago did you send the bloods?'

'Five minutes.'

Henry nodded. 'Get on to Pathology. Ask how long before we get some results.'

Amelia sped off.

The nurse in charge of Emergency appeared at his elbow. 'Anything I can do for you, Henry?'

'Afternoon, Jolene. Yes, please. Open up that LP set you have ready. I'll do it in this small suture theatre if it's free. And grab a consent form for Lulu, thanks.'

Jolene sped off. He turned to Lulu. Her eyes were wide and scared.

'What's wrong with Jake?'

Henry hated this part. 'My first thought is infection. I'd like to do a lumbar puncture. That's placing a needle into the fluid around his spine. He has to curl up for the procedure so the vertebrae open and I can draw off some spinal fluid from the space. It would help if you cuddle his neck and shoulders while we do it. You up for that?'

Lily nodded emphatically. 'I'm up for that.'

Henry smiled at her. 'I never doubted it.'

She brushed that aside. 'So? What are you thinking, Henry?'

'Could be just a nasty virus, but also a bacterial or viral illness which could possibly have progressed to create swelling in the brain. We won't know that until we get the results back from the spinal fluid.'

'How long does that take?'

'A while. But we can start treatment after we do the procedure, not before, or we might mask the organism before we can isolate it.'

'Will he be all right?'

'Results say how we can treat it. But I think Jake has all the symptoms of meningitis. Except maybe a sore throat.'

'He had that this morning, but I thought it was left over from last week.' Lulu pulled on the stud in her lip. 'But you can treat this?'

'Yes. As soon as we get that lumbar puncture done. In case it's bacterial we'll give him antibiotics directly into his vein. He already has the cannula, so he doesn't have to have another drip. We'll add IV fluids to prevent some dehydration through that. And if he gets breathless we'll be giving him some oxygen through a face mask, so he doesn't have to breathe too hard and fast to get what he needs.'

'Will he be in the children's ward?'

'In a day or so. For now, I'll send him to Intensive Care so I can monitor his heart and blood pressure more closely. He'll be in hospital for a few days to a week if all goes well.'

Lulu nodded. 'Is it contagious? Should I bring Jackson in to get checked?'

Henry touched her shoulder again. 'If he's well, he's fine. If he's not well, bring him in.'

Lulu nodded. She was doing a lot of that, pale and shocked by Jake's rapid decline. But her sensible questions had Henry amazed at her composure.

'I thought they'd got over what they had the other day.'

'This is probably something different.'

The charge nurse pulled back the curtain and asked Lulu to sign the consent while another nurse and an orderly unlocked Jake's bed and began to move it out through the curtains. They had a plan and everything would happen fast.

Henry explained the risks and reasons for the lumbar puncture and when Lulu had signed the form they followed Jake's bed down into another, walled room with a door, not just curtains. Once they were inside, the nurse shut the door.

Nadia was waiting when they left the treatment room, and Henry felt that little skip his heart made every time he saw her unexpectedly. He smiled and she smiled back, but there was something he didn't have time to interpret in her eyes.

She made up for that when she handed Lulu the overnight backpack and Henry the packed lunches.

'You haven't eaten,' she said to him. 'Put them in a fridge somewhere.'

His stomach rumbled in agreement.

'Thank you.'

She nodded, hugged a grateful Lulu and left them.

Lulu followed Henry to Intensive Care, where Jake had been moved, lying flat after the lumbar puncture. Henry sat Lulu down in a small tearoom, put the food from Nadia in the fridge for later and made the stressed Lulu a cup of tea.

'The fluid that I took from the space in Jake's spinal looked cloudy, Lulu, which suggests an infection we need to treat. His blood tests confirmed that.'

Lulu paled even further, if that was possible. 'So, meningitis?'

'Yes. Likely. We've started the antibiotics and if Jake shows more symptoms of swelling around his brain we may add steroids to his medications to reduce symptoms.'

Lulu sobbed once. 'Swelling around the brain is bad, isn't it.'

'Not good.' He pushed her cup closer. 'There are risks, Lulu.'

Her eyes were wide and terrified. 'Like what?

He didn't look away, saying softly, 'Worst case scenario, it could cause damage.'

Lulu's eyes widened even further in horror. 'You mean brain damage?'

'It's a risk, but not yet. I have to add there's also a chance of hearing loss, but we're not there yet either. We brought him in early, within a few hours of the first symptoms, so Jake's got every chance of being back home with you in a few days to a week with no problems.'

Lulu closed her eyes. 'Okay.' She gulped. 'Not to worry about that today. Got it.'

But Henry could see the swallowing of horror as she breathed.

He stepped in and hugged her to his chest. Her body shook with distress. Single parents did it even harder, which made him think of Nadia and Katie and the fact that they didn't have arms to hold them.

He stepped back, letting his arms fall. 'We're on this, Lulu. He'll have the best care. It's what we do here.' He gestured to the ward. 'You can't have a bed here, but you can sit in a chair a lot of the time. And when he goes to the children's ward you can stay with him overnight there, in a bed. Okay?'

She clutched his sleeve. 'You'll watch him when I'm not here, won't you, Henry?'

'He'll be watched. Either me or my residents or registrar will be coming a lot and the nurses here are experts at critical care nursing. He'll sleep for a few hours now. If you need to go home and see your mother, now's a good time. Give me your mobile number and I'll text you right now, so you have my number.'

Quickly, he entered her details and texted *Henry* to her phone. It pinged straight away.

Lulu blew out a big breath, looking at the text. 'Thank you. I really appreciate this.'

'You're welcome. You go home now and reassure them. Update your mother and Jackson, and I'll sit here for a bit while I write up my notes.'

Henry watched her go, aching for her distress, but he would do everything in his power to get Jake home to her, undamaged.

Then his eyes were drawn back to the boy lying so pale against the white sheets. Jake lay deeply asleep, moaning softly every now and then, and Henry suspected his headache caused him distress. The boy's chest rose and fell with the rapid breathing and Henry glanced at the monitor to see the telltale sign of desaturation in the pulse oximeter numbers that had come down just a little.

He looked up at the nurses' station and instantly the nurse who was caring for Jake appeared. On the ball, he thought approvingly. The staff everywhere in this hospital were top-notch.

'Thanks, Helen. I'll order a dose of IV Panadol for pain, and see if you can put some nasal prongs on if Jake will tolerate them. If not, then a mask at two litres a minute.'

The nurse nodded. 'To bring his respirations down a bit and his O2 saturation up.'

Henry smiled. 'Yes, and can you make sure his mother, Lulu, is looked after and can come in any time?'

'Of course.' She turned and left to collect the medication and pass on the orders.

Before she could get out of earshot he added, 'Phone my registrar Amelia immediately if there are any concerns and me if there's any delay getting onto her.'

'Will pass that on.'

Henry would document all those orders in the patient notes, but it never hurt to back up the orders with verbal ones as well. Sometimes staff became so busy they didn't get a chance to read the latest notes until it was too late.

He wasn't having that happen to Jake or any of his patients.

Henry stayed with Jake for an hour, not seeing any improvement despite all his positive vibes, and when Lulu came back he left her there. He ate the delayed lunch in the fridge that Nadia had brought, ate hers too as he hoped she'd expected and then took himself to the children's ward for a round.

Everything was fine. He could go. Had to.

He started to walk home, worrying about Jake and the stricken Lulu and wishing he could talk to someone.

Friday had proved too busy for the spot of consolidating Henry had hoped to achieve after work. He'd been thinking about an impromptu invitation to Friday night pizza, relaxing in his place or hers, but in the end he made it home and fell into bed at ten that night.

He took himself to the gym on Saturday morning because his morning runs with Malachi Madden were weekdays only and he needed to burn off nervous energy. For some reason, he felt that today's family visit could be a pivotal moment in his budding relationship with Nadia.

On the blokey side, he enjoyed the dawn outings with Malachi's amusingly blunt pronouncements as they ran along the foreshore paths. Malachi and his family were coming this afternoon for the barbecue, he thought as he pumped iron at the gym, and he enjoyed the clatter of lots of children. He'd been looking forward to Simon's barbecue for days.

And chauffeuring Nadia. His first tenuous inclusion in Nadia and Katie's world. Musing on the progress of his pursuit of Nadia Hargraves, because that was what it was becoming—a pursuit. She certainly wasn't doing any of the chasing.

At least he'd discovered she found him attractive. Relief there. He laughed at himself. Marco would be rolling his eyes. Henry didn't believe he was gorgeous but still, it was better than Nadia saying he left her cold.

He still believed the main stumbling block was rooted in the past. Maybe her dad, who Henry really wanted to meet now, to suss what all that was about. And maybe try to ask her about the dead husband with the roving eye. But he needed time to draw it out of her.

All in all, perhaps they had progressed, though not in the easy manner Henry had hoped for.

He had a date on the weekend, which was what he'd been aiming for. And she had said dinner would be fun. And perhaps when they had Catherine in the car, not the planned inclusion on his little family day out, she could prove a bonus. He liked Catherine, and knew she often minded Katie when Nadia had to work out of usual times. Maybe she would offer to babysit for them to go to dinner. Yes. All in all, lunch had worked out well, if not very well.

Fifteen minutes before the departure for Simon's house his phone rang, and his stomach sank.

Amelia's strained voice, requesting assistance. One of his small patients had relapsed and his registrar felt concerned enough to want an on-site consult.

Of course he would go. Now. As soon as he explained to Nadia.

When he knocked at the ground floor, Katie opened the door. She stared up at him, her little face alight with expectation.

'Dr Henry! We're going to Auntie Bella's in your car!'

Oh, dear heaven.

'Darling Katie, how are you? Is Mummy there?'

Nadia stepped from the bathroom with a hairbrush in one hand and a curve to her lips that made him want to kiss her lovely mouth. Her hair gleamed and face looked serene as she smiled. 'Hello, Henry, you're early.'

'Sadly, I'll be late.'

'Oh.' A cooler voice.

'I'm sorry. I've just been called back to the hospital. I'll have to meet you at Simon's later. They've just phoned from the children's ward.'

'Of course.' He saw something he didn't want to see cross her face. But she smiled carefully and nodded. 'Sure, we'll see you there.'

He looked down at Katie's frowning face. 'I'm sorry, sweetheart.'

'Aren't we going in your car now?'

'Next time. A little boy is sick and I need to

go to the hospital to see him. That means I can't come with you yet.'

'Like Uncle Simon does sometimes?'

He nodded. 'Yes. But I have to go now.'

Nadia said, 'Of course. We hope the child gets better soon.'

When he still stood there, she waved him away. 'Go. I know you're in a hurry.'

He blinked. 'Thanks. Sorry about that. See you.'

'Sure,' she said. 'Shut the door, Katie.'

By the time Henry made it to Simon's barbecue he had no doubt that if any of the food was left, his would be plated and covered with foil.

The first person he saw was little Katie. Her bright green eyes narrowed on him. 'You missed the barbecue.'

As the words left the child's mouth, Nadia appeared behind her with her tote in her hand. She said calmly, 'How is your patient, Henry?'

'Improving, thank you.'

'I'm glad for them.' She said to Katie, 'Doctors have to be there for their patients, Katie. When people are sick, that's more important than everything else.'

Henry frowned. The words were basically correct, but something was off, and Henry felt the sinking in his gut deepen.

'More important than us?' In surprise, Katie

swung her face between Henry and Nadia. Henry knew exactly what Nadia was going to say, and he jumped in.

'Nobody is more important than you and your mummy, Katie. But sometimes I have to miss out on fun times even when I don't want to.'

'Yes,' said Nadia neutrally. She gave him one of those unconvincing smiles he was beginning to dislike intensely. 'We're just about to leave. Malachi and Lisandra have gone. Gran's tired and my sister has finally noticed she's heavily pregnant. She needs a nap.'

'Of course,' he said, cursing under his breath. 'Do you have plans for tomorrow?'

'Let's just see how it pans out,' she said vaguely as her family drifted out behind her, congregating towards the door, where they all hugged and kissed.

Bella came up to Henry. 'Welcome! I'll just see this lot out.'

Everyone greeted him, but in this instance he felt like an outsider. It was something he didn't like to feel. In fact, it made him feel like the ostracised kid in the mended clothes with no dad, the one he'd been at school. Especially when weighed against the sense of inclusion he'd savoured the last time this group of people had gathered.

Simon turned to Henry. 'Sorry you missed out on lunch.'

Everyone left and Bella returned. 'There's a full

plate in the fridge for you. You should eat before the salad goes limp.'

Simon touched his wife's shoulder. 'I'll sort Henry and you'll go and rest.' Henry felt his friend's sympathetic gaze on him. 'I'll make sure he gets his lunch. Henry and I will have a very comfortable afternoon doing blokey stuff.'

Bella said, 'But…'

'And we'll empty the dishwasher now it's finished and listen for Kai if he wakes.'

As this domestic jostle progressed, it dawned on Henry that he was so late that even the dishwasher had finished its cycle after the event. He'd missed it all. Completely.

Five minutes later, when they were both sitting at the table, Simon with a coffee and Henry carving into a reheated tender wagyu with lashings of potato bake, Simon said, 'Bad luck on that timing, mate.'

Henry put his fork down and stared glumly at his plate. 'I think I may have gone back four steps.'

Simon sipped his coffee thoughtfully. 'At least four.'

He didn't get it. 'What am I supposed to do? This is my job. That's why I studied and trained. I'm a doctor who is called into work. It's what I am.'

'Finished wallowing?'

Simon's soft voice had Henry's chin up in no time. He wasn't wallowing.

The aggravating man opposite had his hand up in amusement. 'I get that. It's what you do. What we do.' He paused. 'Listen to me. We love our jobs, but if we want to keep the women we love you need to understand that our work is not who we are.'

And how did that pan out?

'I'm pretty sure Nadia wouldn't want me to not care about my patients.'

And that hadn't sounded sulky like a child, Henry thought, wishing the words back. He really had worked himself up and he didn't like it.

'I'm sure Nadia admires your dedication,' Simon said dryly, 'but she won't be admiring from up close. As for missing lunch, today wasn't a big event, just a little family barbecue. There was no tragedy or disruption to anybody because you weren't here.'

Ouch. Henry didn't like the sound of that, but had to accept it was true. He put down his knife and fork, his appetite satisfied and his heart heavy.

Simon wasn't finished with the tough love. 'But if it had been, say…a formal event with Nadia all dressed to go, and your resident called you with exactly the same phone conversation, would you go?'

'Yes. Of course.' He heard the words before he thought it through.

Simon nodded. 'I applaud you for it. But if there is something budding between you and Nadia, that lack of forethought might just cost you a family.'

Henry shook his head. 'People marry doctors. They're happy. This can't be right.'

'Your dilemmas were mine four years ago,' Simon said.

'What am I supposed to do?'

Simon rubbed his chin. 'Talk to Nadia. Find out what she thinks. I can't help you there.'

Henry shook his head. 'I thought there was a good thing happening here, Simon.'

'I'm seeing that. And I can share that Nadia cast more than a few glances towards the door today. She looked disappointed when you weren't there.'

That was something.

'Do you think it's too late?'

Simon held up his hands. 'Over my pay grade as your mentor-slash-buddy. Depends how hard you want to try.' He stood and walked to the fridge. Came back with two beers, handed one to Henry. The silence lengthened between them. Simon patiently sipped.

Henry said slowly, 'When I thought I might have to fight for Nadia, I thought it would be against another man, not against my work.'

'Hmm. Does it change how you feel about her?'

Henry's whole being rebelled. 'No, of course not. Just makes me depressed.'

'Oh, spare me that too,' Simon murmured, and Henry had to smile.

He had sounded pathetic. Maybe he could explain. 'Not something I talk about, but my dad left when I was seven. My mum worked really, really hard to keep a roof over our heads. She died young.'

Simon said quietly, 'I'm sorry.'

'Other people have it worse.' Henry took a sip of his beer and put it down again. 'A big part of my work is making sure that I have a solid base. When I do find a partner for life, no way will she ever have to work like my mother did. She'd never be left destitute.' He looked up at Simon. 'If it was Nadia... I would keep her and Katie safe.'

Simon put his beer down and sat back in his chair, a perplexed frown on his face. 'Admirable sentiments and sympathy for the young Henry. But saying that out loud to Nadia could get you thrown out. Which century are you living in?'

Henry blinked.

Simon laughed and waved an apologetic hand. 'Nadia is an independent woman. Self-sufficient. Doesn't need you to provide, because she can meet every material need she and Katie have.'

The words were colder on his skin than the beer he rested his hand against. It took a few moments for them to sink in past the gooseflesh.

Oh, damn. He sat back. He'd been so stupid.

In London, sixteen thousand kilometres away,

he'd been so focused on achieving his career goals so he could nurture and care for his future partner, like he'd wanted to nurture and care for his mother, he'd dropped reality.

While he'd been in London, his memory of Nadia had been based on the beautiful but fragile young widow in a wheelchair with a premature baby, the mysterious woman he'd been attracted to at first sight. He hadn't been able to care for her five years ago because she had her family. But he had built a fantasy world around the whimsical possibility that he might in the future.

In fact, she still had her family. She had herself. She didn't need him.

A lot of that self-loathing must have crossed his face because Simon said, 'Before you take yourself off to drown your sorrows, listen to me.'

He dragged himself out of despair and looked up.

'Women have other needs than a roof over their heads, though that is essential too. If you want to be a part of Nadia's and Katie's lives, be an equal partner and parent. They need your presence more than they need you to provide anything.'

And how did he do that?

'Not much of me to go around. I work ten to fifteen hours a day. I've been stupid. Patriarchal. Maybe I don't have anything they need.'

Simon looked at his empty stubby as if it had

let him down. Sighing, he said, 'Yes, you do. You have you.'

Henry grunted. Pushed away the small bottle in front of him. This was bad.

'I should just back off. This isn't going to work.'

'And you heard me say she cast more than a few glances towards the door today.'

'Sure.'

'She did. You're in a tough place, Henry. First dates and starting out as a new consultant. Finding your feet and making connections with colleagues. Moving up. If you want Nadia, you're going to have to figure out the balance. We can't put our wives and families on hold whenever it suits us.'

Simon finished his beer. 'And that's enough about you.' He shook himself as if it was all too much. 'I want football. The Broncos are playing South Sydney at Suncorp Stadium in five minutes.'

Henry held up his hands. 'I'm done.'

Simon had given him some advice. If he wanted to pursue Nadia, he needed to figure this out for himself. There were very capable doctors a few suburbs away, working at other hospitals. Maybe he needed a bigger team.

He sat back. Thought that through. He knew of several good paeds. He could cultivate some backup.

CHAPTER THIRTEEN

Nadia

DRIVING HOME FROM BELLA'S, Nadia glanced in the rear-view mirror. 'Katie's gone to sleep already,' she said to her grandmother.

'Lucky Katie,' said Catherine and put her hand up to cover her yawn.

Nadia smiled. 'You'll be having your own little nana nap in fifteen minutes. The traffic's heavy, so it will take us a bit to get home.'

They drove for a few more minutes until they stopped at a traffic light behind a long line of cars. Catherine shifted in her seat and faced her. *Here it comes*, thought Nadia, heroically not sighing out loud.

'So? Are you going to forgive the man?'

And that would be Gran, not beating around the bush.

'I'm still too annoyed to think about it.'

'He looked like someone popped a paper bag in front of his face when you left.'

'He probably didn't even notice the time while at work,' said Nadia. 'Just like Dad. Too busy being that consultant.' When Catherine didn't say anything, she went on. 'I'm more angry with myself. I knew this was going to happen. And yet I opened myself up to disappointment. Katie was disappointed.'

Yes. Definitely more annoyed with herself. And, sadly, definitely disappointed with her idea of Henry.

'But still annoyed with Henry,' said Catherine.

'Oh, yes.'

'The man has a dilemma, you know.'

His problem, thought Nadia, feeling snarky.

'Well, I don't. I'm not having that life. Lovely man, lovely fairy tale. But, in reality, I want a man who's there for me.'

Catherine huffed. 'Oh, for goodness' sake, Nadia, stop. What man is there for you now? What perfect paragon is going to meet all your needs in exactly the way you want?'

Oh, dear, Gran was on a roll, thought Nadia with an inner wince. Thankfully, the lights turned green to go and she could watch the road and avoid those all-seeing eyes.

'If you don't start accepting people aren't perfect, then you will always be alone. It will become harder and harder to connect with someone who could be your life partner.'

Ouch. Gloves off, Gran. It would even be painful if she hadn't heard it before.

'Take second best, you mean?'

Gran growled.

'Okay.' Carefully, she said, 'You're saying I just forget that this was the first time we actually looked ahead? A proper planned outing. That he had advance notice for.' She really didn't want to say *date*. 'And just forget he didn't turn up until it was all over?'

'Yes,' said Catherine simply. 'He's a new consultant. His patient was sick. He's never held this position before. He has to find a way to arrange his life balance.'

'All perfectly reasonable, even admirable, for a doctor. But not my dream person, and not someone I plan to pin my life on.'

Catherine pushed on. 'Give him a bit of leeway to make mistakes.'

'You think today was a mistake? He didn't realise?' She could hear the incredulity in her voice and toned it down. Said quietly, firmly. 'I think it's the beginning of a pattern.'

'Of course you do. You've been hyperalert for traits of your father since you started dating.'

There was a silence then. Nadia feeling cross with her grandmother now and no doubt Gran struggling not to say what Nadia knew she wanted to say. *And you married the wrong man because of that.*

More calmly, Gran said, 'If I know Simon, he'll have given him sensible advice already.'

Nadia thought about her big brother-in-law—a mentor Henry looked up to, the man married to her sister. A little of her ire seeped away. Yes, Simon would have advice. Could it help? Would Henry listen?

Catherine said, 'Give him another chance.'

Nadia blew out a big breath. She enjoyed Henry's company and his attention. Found herself thinking of Henry when she shouldn't. The man was intruding and if he wasn't going to be there it had to stop. Stubbornly, she asserted, 'An over-committed consultant is not what I want for Katie and me.'

Gran snorted. 'Well, pull up your big girl panties and tell him. If that's the big problem, don't whistle down the wind until you've had a chance to tell him why.'

Thankfully, they were just pulling into the underground car park of the units. Katie woke with the sound of the rumbling roller door. 'Home,' she said sleepily.

'Home, darling,' Nadia said. And that was the thing. More than anything, she didn't want Katie to have a part-time father.

When she'd gone to bed last night Nadia had listened to her relaxation track to calm down and in response she'd had a good night's sleep.

So when Henry phoned the next morning, she knew it was him because she'd swapped in his new number for his old. Funny that. His old number had been in her phone all the time since Katie had been born. Because, yes, he'd been so very good when Katie had been in the NICU, so she smiled and answered.

Thought about her grandmother's words. Maybe she would give Henry somewhere between one and four chances.

Before he could say anything, she said, 'Good morning, Henry. Happy Sunday.'

There was a moment's silence at the other end of the phone as if she'd interrupted his prepared speech. She smiled. Good—got him off-balance instead of her.

After just a beat he said, 'Happy Sunday, Nadia. Would you and Katie like to go for breakfast at Greenmount Surf Club this morning? And the markets are on at Coolangatta. I thought you might like to walk through there after?'

That did sound lovely.

'Thank you, Henry. I've been meaning to get to the markets for ages. Hadn't realised it was the second Sunday today. What time were you thinking of leaving?'

'Whenever you're both ready.'

She glanced at the clock. Seven-thirty.

'Half an hour?'

'I'll be at your front door at eight.

* * *

Henry arrived promptly at eight. Possibly a few minutes before. This time Nadia opened the door for him.

Before she could say hello, he said, 'I'm sorry about yesterday, Nadia. I'll try to do better in the future.'

And that just took the wind right out of her sails.

'Okay, Henry. And I'll try to give you some leeway. But understand that my childhood meant being stood up by my father at important times. Every time. I'm not planning on doing that for the rest of my life.'

'Noted,' he said, and cautiously both smiled at the other.

'Right,' she said, 'I'll just grab my backpack.'

Katie ignored him as she played with her doll in the corner—scolded the painted face, probably for being late. Nadia thought with a smile that she was mimicking her mother, like she normally was.

'Come on, Katie, Dr Henry's here.'

Katie bounced up with her doll under her arm. She crossed the room to Henry. Tilted her head up at him. 'Mummy said we're going in your car this morning. Is that true?' She didn't look convinced.

Nadia had to suppress the smile. Poor Henry had two women on his back.

He crouched down to Katie's height. 'Yes,

FIONA MCARTHUR   131

Katie. I'm sorry for yesterday. I borrowed a booster seat off Uncle Simon. So I've got a car seat in the back of my car already.'

Katie skipped up and down. 'You have?' Which was just what Nadia was thinking. She'd planned to grab Katie's from the back of her own car on the way through the garage.

Henry glanced over his shoulder at her. 'I did.'

Nadia raised her brows in ironic approval while Katie tilted her head in enquiry. 'Do you have an iPad behind the seat?'

Nadia grinned at Henry's sudden freeze. 'Um… no. No, I don't.'

'Mummy does. And I sing songs while the grown-ups talk in the front.'

Nadia bit her lip to stop the laugh.

Unfazed, Henry agreed, 'I'll have to get one.'

Katie picked up her doll. 'Then I'm ready.'

Breakfast was easy and fun. Greenmount Surf Club overlooked the waves and the sun beat down on the sand in front of them while gulls squabbled over morsels found at the edge of the water.

Katie had been given a pack of crayons and paper by the staff and was happily drawing stick figures on a sunny day.

She and Henry had fallen into a desultory ramble of comments and observations and Nadia realised that, despite all her protestations of being happily single, she had desperately missed adult male conversation. And Henry's company was pretty darn special.

And maybe the admiring looks whenever Henry glanced her way were very nice too. Which was often. And very warming.

'Looking for anything special at the markets?' Henry asked.

'Little things for a Miss…' She spelled out Katie's age. 'Next month.'

Henry's smile made her catch her breath. White teeth, sexy lips curved and his dark brown eyes crinkled with delight. 'Are you having a… P-A-R-T-Y?' He spelled out the word. 'May I come?'

'Yes. At Bella's with three extra visitors coming.'

'What time?' he asked.

She tilted her head and narrowed her eyes at him. 'Eleven. I'll see you there.'

She actually thought he gulped, and she softened. 'Or not. It's entirely up to you, Henry.'

'I will do everything in my power,' he said. And, strangely, she believed him.

The markets proved fun, but by the time they'd finished, Katie's head drooped and she fell asleep even before Henry drove them back to the units.

'I'm going to put Katie to bed for a little nap with her doll. Ernestine's tired,' she said.

'You could carry Ernestine, and I could carry Katie up for you?'

And didn't that just make her smile. *Oh, Henry, you are a charmer.*

'If you do that, I could offer you a cup of tea.' Because she wasn't ready to say goodbye to him yet either.

CHAPTER FOURTEEN

Henry

HENRY CONSIDERED HIMSELF very fortunate to be sitting one down from Nadia on her three-seater couch with the teacups and pretty teapot on the table in front of them.

Katie hadn't woken when Henry put her into bed. Feeling Katie's cheek against his shoulder and her small hands around his neck had been the most amazing sensation. He'd been surprised how fortunate he'd felt to be trusted by the child and her mother.

He'd lifted kids before, many times, but not one he'd known since birth. A little girl he found himself growing more fond of every second, and little Katie's freely given trust and snuggle-ability made a strange protective urge surge unexpectedly inside him.

He'd watched as Nadia slipped her daughter's shoes off, tucked her doll—Ernestine, Henry reminded himself—beside her and covered her up.

It was almost as if he was a part of her family. Nadia's family.

Dear heaven, was this where he wanted to be?

Now, Katie's bedroom door stood ajar, which kept their voices low, and in the background, country music played softly as the open veranda door allowed the sea breeze to flutter the curtains.

'You can pull up the tab at your end of the lounge, you know, to give you a footrest,' Nadia said.

Lazily, Henry raised his brows at her. She demonstrated and once she'd kicked off her blue sandals her feet were bare and suspended above the tiles.

His gut twisted at the sight of her bare toes. So exposed. Fragile. Womanly toes. He moistened suddenly dry lips.

'You have beautiful feet.'

'Thank you,' she said.

He so dearly wanted to cup them in his hands.

'I give a great foot rub.' He had a sudden, very graphic fantasy of lifting one slender leg and kissing those feet. His body stirred.

She turned her head and quirked an eyebrow at him. 'Do you?'

'So I've been told.' It had been his mum, but he wouldn't share that.

Or maybe he could. Maybe he should. He forced himself.

'My mum said that. Dad left when I was seven.

She worked really hard.' He wanted to push those memories of his exhausted mother away, but perhaps Nadia needed to know. 'Sometimes I'd rub her feet for her after work.'

Nadia stared at him. The glorious blue of her eyes went so soft his breath caught. But he wanted understanding, not sympathy, so he changed the subject.

'Anyway, dear Nadia, one day I'd like to rub your feet.' He watched as her sympathy turned to something else as he imagined again holding Nadia's slim feet in his hands and let it show on his face.

Her cheeks pinked and her mouth curved. With her response, instantly his body stirred until he had to force cooling thoughts—icy showers, polar bears, Nadia being scared. That worked to cool him. Not tonight. But soon.

'But…' back under control '… I won't say no to the footrest.'

She murmured, 'And I won't say no to some future foot rub.'

Henry glanced back at her toes, mesmerised. She had small slender feet with perfect nails painted pink at the tips. There was something private about those toes that he'd been allowed to see. He couldn't remember feeling this at home with a woman. Ever.

He tried his own footrest and took the weight

off his legs like a…husband? Leaned back and closed his eyes.

'All we need now is a movie and some popcorn for the perfect Sunday afternoon,' he murmured, to lighten the unexpectedly heavy impact of that thought.

Nadia laughed. Her voice was a whisper of dancing notes in the quiet room. 'That does sound relaxing. Do you watch many movies, Henry?'

He opened his eyes. 'None in the day. At night, when I can't sleep, sometimes.'

She leaned with her cheek on her knuckles, elbow resting on the side arm of the sofa as she watched him. 'What sort of movies do you watch?'

'Prefer old ones.' His drowsiness receded. 'But anything that's on, really.'

'Yes, but what's your favourite?'

He closed his eyes to think because he couldn't while he watched her. Thought about what he enjoyed. 'Old Westerns. Clint Eastwood. Saloon girls and rough, tough ranchers.'

He heard her laugh softly and his lips curved. He loved that sound. Could easily love her, he realised. That hadn't taken long. Damn. He was already in too deep for his precarious position.

'You like romance and bromance. I love it.' She was on another page. As usual.

He blinked. Bromance? Where had that come

from? he thought, and then remembered the conversation before his own internal revelation.

'Um…yes. What about you?'

'Rom-coms.' Her eyes sparkled and he sat straighter in the chair, reducing the angle.

She had a faraway look in her eyes and a reminiscent smile on her lovely face that he wanted to see when she thought about him. 'Ones that make me laugh and then make me sad and then smile again. And yes, the old ones are fab, just like your Westerns.'

Pulling the chair out of its recliner mode, he put his feet back on the floor. *Ground yourself, mate.* Because he just wanted to reach sideways and pull her to him.

'Name one.'

She shrugged. '*French Kiss* with Meg Ryan. *Sleepless in Seattle. The Princess Bride. Notting Hill.*'

'Nope. Don't know any of them. But the kiss one sounds promising.' He fancied a bit of French kissing.

'Seriously? Never watched any of them?' Her eyes widened and he smiled. She'd missed his innuendo.

'Cross my heart.' He mimed the action.

'Well.' She put her own footrest down with a click and stood. 'Stay there. You need educating. I'll just put the popcorn maker on.'

'Please do.' Suddenly, he wasn't sleepy. At all. He stood too. 'But let me help.'

She waved him back. 'No. It's a small kitchen and I'll get flustered with your big body in there with me.'

Hell, yeah.

He grinned. 'I'd like that.' He loomed as much as he could without crowding her.

'I'm sure you would.' Primly, she pointed to a wall but with laughter in her eyes as she moved towards the kitchen.

He didn't sit. Instead, he shifted so he could lean on the wall near the kitchen with his arms crossed across his chest and watched her economical movements as she pulled a small red contraption out of the cupboard and put it on the granite bench. Plugged it in.

Watched her lithe yet luscious body stretch up to a top cupboard, her breasts outlined as she stretched the bodice of the lacy shirt and lifted out a container of rattling beads. His mouth turning dry. Hungry. Not for the popcorn.

She must have felt him watching.

'Haven't you ever seen someone make popcorn?'

'Not like this.' And he wasn't talking about the roasting. Nothing like this. His mouth a desert, he searched for an answer. 'Maybe in the movie theatre.'

'Only in the movie theatre? Didn't your mum make you popcorn?'

He didn't answer. Didn't want to go there again this afternoon and kill the magic.

Finally, he said, 'No. Do you put oil in there?'

'Not with the machine. You do if you put it in a pot on the stove, though I did read they turn out better if you don't.'

She concentrated on the task at hand and he could see she was only half listening to him. Good. Easier to watch and savour. He knew nothing about the intricacies of popping corn. But maybe it was his new favourite pastime. Absolute fave. That would be watching Nadia make popcorn. She took about a quarter of a cup of bright yellow corn kernels from the cannister and poured them in the top of the machine and turned it on. She looked quite satisfied with herself and he smiled.

'What movie are we going to watch?'

'I think *French Kiss*. Kevin Kline does it for me.'

Now that she was just waiting, he decided it should be safe to crowd her a little.

'Yeah? Well… You do it for me.' He moved in and stood close behind her as she faced the popcorn maker. Slid his arms around her waist. 'I'd like to do it for you, but I don't think we're quite at that stage,' he murmured, his voice amused.

More softly and seriously, he whispered, 'But I would like to kiss you.'

She spun slowly, her body turning within his arms, thankfully not pushing him away, until she faced him and looked up. Still in his circle. So close. A teasing womanly smile tilting that gorgeous mouth.

Very softly, very near to his mouth, she whispered back, 'If I was honest, Henry, I'd have to say I'd like to kiss you too.'

His heartrate spiked. 'Fortunate.' His voice coming out deep and low. Breathing in her scent. He leaned across the tiny distance between them to brush her mouth oh-so-gently with his.

Heaven help him, her lips were so soft. His arms tightened, pulling her close against his body. So warm. So soft.

Behind them, the first corn kernel popped and he felt her lips smile against his.

The kiss deepened and he was lost in the heat. The taste of her mouth. His tongue nudged against softness and she opened to him, offering her breath, herself.

Henry groaned and kissed Nadia until his head swam, not demanding but savouring, learning, losing himself in her, with her, entwining and tangled and tormented. A whole world of sensation which was new and wonderful, even for their first time.

By the time he stepped back, the last pops from

the machine were sporadic and Nadia's eyes were shut. Her breasts rose and fell, rose and fell with her rapid breathing and he savoured the feel of her soft body squashed against his.

Henry leaned past her and switched the machine off at the wall, with no idea how to turn it off at the control panel and not really interested enough to ask.

He came back to her and smoothed her velvet cheek with a reverential finger, watching her face, the roses in her cheeks, the thoroughly kissed blush of her mouth.

Nadia blew out a slow breath and opened her eyes. Her lips curved, slightly swollen, pink and delicious.

'Well, Henry Oliver,' she whispered, 'it seems that's another thing you do very, very well.'

He felt his smile stretch. 'Ditto, dear Nadia. I could kiss you until the whole world was full of popcorn.'

CHAPTER FIFTEEN

Nadia

OH, MY. NADIA felt like fanning her face. Henry was just too dangerous. In fact, she was feeling a tad daring herself right at this moment.

The silence stretched and she realised the popping had stopped.

'Oh, popcorn's ready. Don't want it to burn.' Inane but better than the silence.

She spun to see the popcorn maker. It lay full and silent.

'I turned it off,' was his laconic response.

How had she missed that? She knew how.

'Did you? Oh. When?'

'Just a second ago. Before you opened your eyes.' His brown eyes were watching hers with a decidedly masculine appreciation. 'Can we do that again?'

'We don't need more popcorn,' she said, pretending to misunderstand him, and spun to lift the lid. 'We've probably got thirty minutes of movie watching time before Katie wakes and wants to sit between us.'

He stepped back to give her room, but didn't leave the kitchen. Leant back against the doorway in that pose he seemed to like. Tall, arms folded, watching.

'Does that mean we get to snuggle on the couch until she does?'

That didn't sound too bad.

'Maybe.'

'And *French Kiss*,' he said. 'Definitely *French Kiss*.'

She laughed. 'Of course you're talking about the movie. I'll get right on that.'

She had no doubt that her cheeks had flamed red. And she wanted to lift her fingers to her lips because oh, my, she could still feel his oh-so-sexy mouth on hers. Her belly still jumped and writhed too, and her hands felt empty without the hold she'd had on Henry's muscular back. It was very lucky that Katie was in the other room, keeping her mother just a little bit sane.

'Do you want something to drink?'

'Cold water would be good,' he said. 'I'm feeling a little warm…' He waved his palm back and forth as if creating a breeze, like she'd wanted to do moments ago. His eyes twinkled. 'Really no idea why.'

'Right,' she said as she lined up two glasses from the cupboard and took down two bowls for the popcorn. Though she didn't need to keep their bowls separate as they'd already plastered their mouths against each other. Dipping in and eating the same popcorn wasn't going to make a difference. Thoughtfully, she put one dish back.

'You put the popcorn in the bowl. I'll fill the water and find the movie.'

Five minutes later, they were settled, no 'Mind the gap' between them. Hips touching, arms brushing, shoulders heated. No gap at all.

As the movie intro began to roll, Henry reached down and took her fingers in his and cupped her hand. Yep, she couldn't help the smile on her face. She looked down at his fingers and the popcorn on the small table and decided maybe they should lift the bowl into her lap. For safety. For the popcorn. And for her.

She reached and juggled until she had it settled. 'Holding hands does make it awkward.'

He shrugged. Dug into the popcorn. 'Bringing that popcorn closer is a great idea.'

By the time Katie pulled open her door, rubbing her eyes with her fists, they were engrossed in the movie. Henry had laughed more than a few times at the witty repartee, and she loved the sound of his deep laugh as much as she had the first time she'd heard it. Maybe more.

'Hello, darling. Come sit up here.' She patted her

lap. The bowl had been moved for safety a long time ago. 'Henry's watching a movie with me.'

Katie shuffled across and instead of sitting on her mother's lap or at her side, as she had wryly expected, she stood between them and wriggled her body until there was space for three on the lounge like sardines.

Henry met Nadia's eyes over the top of Katie's blonde head as her daughter settled in between the adults. 'This is nice,' he mouthed.

Nadia agreed. Fabulous, but also terrifying. Still, she consoled herself, they were only watching a movie.

And they'd only kissed.

Yeah. Only, huh?

Quite a few times, actually, while the movie ran. But everything would be back to normal and slow down now their chaperone was here.

When the movie was finished and they started *Saving Nemo* for Katie, it proved more fun as the adults chuckled while Katie sat immersed in the movie, occasionally glancing at them as if wondering why they were laughing.

A perfect afternoon.

When it was over Henry stood to help her clear up dropped popcorn from the floor and empty glasses, and slowly her sanity returned.

He tilted his head and suggested, 'Would I be

pushing my luck if I offered takeaway pizza at my house?'

'I think so,' said Nadia quietly. 'It's been a lovely day, Henry. Thank you for taking us out for breakfast and the markets.'

'Watching movies with you and Katie has been the nicest Sunday I've had for a long time,' he said.

Nice. For some reason, she thought of her grandmother and her dislike of *pleasant.* Nadia decided she didn't like *nice* either.

'I hope we do it again,' he said.

His words stole her amusement away. She sucked in a breath.

Shifting her hip back his way until they were touching again, she whispered, 'Henry, you're just the dream man, aren't you?'

'It's what I've been telling you.' He went on, 'Sometimes you are so slow.'

She laughed.

'Now. Come out on a date with me. A real evening date, dressing up, with a proper restaurant. Can you find somebody to mind Katie just for one evening?'

Suddenly, she felt unsure of herself. Her friends-with-benefits thought might be a double-edged sword.

'Gran already offered.'

'Good. How about we go out on Wednesday night? My worrisome patient should be well on the mend by then and I'll arrange call cover with another paediatrician.'

Strangely, she approved of his concern for his patient, even when it meant making her wait a few days, and yes, she could do that. A couple of days to think about it would be a good thing.

He stood. Reached and pulled her up and into his arms. Leaned his face down and kissed her thoroughly until she forgot where she was, any objections and concerns about the future, in those moments of bliss, the world as distant as the weather or the waves outside the window.

Henry eased away, stared into her face and seemed satisfied with what he saw there—probably a gaping fish, the way she felt—and strode to the door.

'Wednesday. I'll pick you up at six. We're going to have drinks and a posh dinner and maybe go dancing.'

'I haven't danced for years.'

He looked smug. 'I'm very good.'

She laughed. Who was this new Henry?

'And you have tickets on yourself.'

'I'm pinning them up there so you can see them and feel reassured I will stop you treading on my toes. My only reason for bragging.'

'Ah, thoughtful of you.'

'I'm nice like that. Then we'll come back to my place and watch the moon rise over the ocean.'

'That does sound amazing.' Getting dressed

up and going out with a man for the first time in years…with Henry. That idea was terrifying and exhilarating. She wasn't sure which emotion was winning. But no strings was good, though Henry hadn't been as eager as she'd expected.

She'd never wanted to risk her heart, and this wasn't a stranger she would see once and never again. This was Henry and she had taken steps to not get in deeper than she wanted.

'Then another day we'll take Katie out.' He grinned at her. 'There are all sorts of fun places we can go to on the Gold Coast. I'd love to spend Sundays with the two of you.'

Before he could say more his phone buzzed quietly, but he didn't answer it. Just texted quickly. Then smiled at Nadia. 'Lucky you were throwing me out. Bye-bye, Katie,' he called, and her daughter looked up from where she was talking to Ernestine about the fishy movie.

He leaned in and kissed Nadia's still sensitive lips very softly before she realised his intention.

Then he was gone before she could kiss him back, his voice trailing behind him. '… I'll see you tomorrow at work.'

As she closed the door, Nadia turned and rested against the hard wood, cool against her back.

Thinking about the day. Thinking about the kiss. And thinking about the trouble she was in if she didn't want to fall for Henry.

CHAPTER SIXTEEN

Henry

HENRY WALKED AWAY from Nadia's door with his phone to his ear. 'I'm on my way. Five minutes.'

The small change he'd made to his callback protocol had worked well. After Simon's insight he'd considered his options. For normal weekends with no concrete plans he'd cover himself, but he'd told his registrar to text first and then ring if he didn't answer within a couple of minutes. Which gave him a chance to extricate himself without blatantly stepping away from Nadia to answer his phone. He still had to attend, that was the job he loved, but his leaving would not be so in her face.

The whole time he walked towards the hospital he ran over the last eight hours of absolute bliss in his head. It really had been the best Sunday afternoon he'd experienced for years. As for his revelation of moving from desiring Nadia to imagining a possible future with her—that was something he couldn't think about now. But it could stay at the back of his mind, along with those delightful memories of kissing Nadia and holding her in his arms.

But all that needed to be put away as he walked through the front entrance to the hospital.

CHAPTER SEVENTEEN

Nadia

WHEN HENRY LEFT, the room felt suddenly empty and colourless.

She persuaded Katie into the bath, where her daughter always made lots of noise, which helped dispel the hollow quiet of the flat. Still unsettled, she wandered aimlessly until she had a shower herself.

It had been a big day and she felt strangely agitated and unable to settle to any of the tasks she usually performed on Sunday evenings for the week ahead.

Eventually sorted for the week, she glanced at the clock and decided she could make dinner and maybe they'd just go to bed early and read.

It was only when Katie, looking adorable in her unicorn pyjamas, was deep in conversation with Ernestine again that Nadia began to feel more like herself. She listened to her daughter, couldn't help smiling, and waited for a pause in the conversation, shaking her head at the chatter.

Finally, Katie drew breath and Nadia asked, 'What would you like for dinner, darling?'

'Pizza.' Her daughter's instant reply made Nadia frown.

Little minx, she must have heard Henry when he'd mentioned pizza earlier. At the time she'd looked so immersed in playing with her doll, Nadia thought wryly.

A good reminder that Katie missed little.

'I could make pizza. On those flatbreads—you like them, don't you? What sort would you like?'

'I like all your pizzas, Mummy.'

Not helpful.

'Well, choose. Pineapple and ham? Pepperoni? Or just cheese and tomato?'

'What sort does Dr Henry like?'

Nadia blinked. Yes, if she'd needed proof that her daughter was aware of everything going on, that was it there. And she'd just got the pesky man out of the forefront of her brain.

'I have no idea what sort of pizza Dr Henry likes, but he's not coming to dinner tonight, so it's about you and me.'

'Ernestine wants to know why he can't come to dinner tonight.'

Oh, spare me.

'Because he's not here.'

Her daughter looked at her as if she were such a silly thing. 'He's just in the flat upstairs.'

As if.

'He had to go to the hospital.' She assumed that was what the text message was all about. And she'd seen enough of Henry Oliver to stop her sleeping tonight, already. She did not need to think about him any more than she had already.

Her belly squirmed. But it had felt good, snuggled up next to Henry and with Katie between them and, judging by his tentative suggestion they do pizza tonight, he'd enjoyed it too.

She could ask him? No doubt about her daughter's feelings on the matter.

Nadia sighed. He probably wasn't back from the hospital anyway.

She watched, as if she were a being taken over by an alien, and her fingers typed a text to Henry.

I'm making small pizzas on flatbread. If you're not busy and you'd like to join us you're welcome. N

The answer came back swiftly.

Have a patient I'm worried about but would love company if you don't mind me dashing away as needed.

And didn't that just epitomise Henry's openness? His disclosure, general though it was, even put a different slant on her aversion to doctors being on call.

Her dad had never made it personal, so she guessed she'd never thought of the reasons he'd left as real dramas for real people. Most likely because of the privacy door that had always been slammed in their faces.

And Henry said he was worried. He wanted company and she had a sudden insight into the loneliness of his life if he didn't have anyone to talk to about those worries. He had put it out there, just like him, despite knowing she could be annoyed if he was called back to the hospital, and even risking her rescinding the dinner invitation.

Strange, she mused, not understanding her own acceptance. Thoughtfully, she texted back.

You have to eat. If you leave, they're small enough to take with you and gobble on the way. N

Sounds amazing. I'm on my way. H

Which was how Henry ended up back on the couch in Nadia's lounge room and she had to admit he looked good there.

Katie had been very satisfied when Henry turned up at the door and couldn't wait to ask, 'What's your favourite pizza, Dr Henry?'

'Whatever your mummy makes, Katie.'

'Me too.'

* * *

The pizza was gone—all types, all variations—
and the conversation had been desultory until
Katie went to bed.

Henry made no move to go and, strangely,
she didn't push him to, and it wasn't even because they'd ended up back on the sofa, hip to
hip, drinking tea.

'You said you were worried about a patient?'
And that was opening herself up to a snub. Any
time she'd tried to ask her father he'd slammed
the privacy and Hippocratic oath at her. She could
remember being crushed enough to let the subject drop.

Henry said, 'I am worried.'

'I know you can't tell me who, but I'm happy
to listen to why you're worried. Maybe it will
help to talk.'

The look he gave her was something she'd
never seen on a man's face before. Certainly not
on Alex's. Her husband had always looked like a
reckless teenager bent on some new adventure,
and their relationship hadn't been this...equal?
Giving? Trusting?

Her heart did a little gallop inside her and her
hand lifted of its own accord and lay warmly on
his thigh for comfort. She'd seen something like
that expression when Katie was sick and Nadia
stroked her brow.

Just for a moment, she could see the young

Henry, not much older than Malachi's twins, needing comfort after his dad walked out. And later, when his mother worked hard. The expression disappeared. But she'd seen the worried child from the past. The boy who cared too much.

A rush of tenderness she hadn't expected made her hand slip from his leg to take his hand in hers to listen.

'This morning this little boy, who is going through chemotherapy, was reasonably well. This afternoon he's critical, confused and in distress. I had to tell his mother he has no immunity at all and at risk of any infection attacking him. I'm afraid he won't survive if he catches something. If that happens, I don't know how I can comfort her. How I can forgive myself for not being able to make him well.'

'Oh, Henry. You comfort her by keeping him alive and giving her hope,' she said quietly, wanting to ease him. 'I'm sure she knows you care. Knows you'll be there when needed. You're a wonderful, compassionate paediatrician, Henry. I saw that myself when Katie was a baby.'

And that was her problem right there. He'd always give to others when needed, even if she needed him, but at this moment it wasn't important.

'You give—be careful you don't give too much. Because you and your skills need to be there for the next little kid and the next.'

'But how? How can I be there and still have what I want for myself in my other life away from work? How do I meld the two worlds?'

Yep. Problem there. And she didn't have the answer.

'I don't know, Henry. I suppose it depends on what you want.'

He turned his head and his gaze held hers. His chocolate-brown eyes suddenly filled with despair. Uncertainty wasn't something she was used to seeing in Henry. And then it was gone. She'd have missed it if their gazes hadn't locked.

He lifted his free hand. 'What we had today. I want this.'

'Except when you get called away.'

'Yes. Except for then.'

'So where do you see this going?'

'I think we could have something good together...if you can take a chance on me.'

She'd wanted to explain. This was her opportunity, but she felt as if she were on a precipice and what they said here could make or break whatever fragile thing there was between them.

'There's a big part of this I want too, Henry.'

'But not all of it?'

'No. I told you about my dad letting us down. We lived with him, loved him, but he wasn't there at all for us. He lived for his work. I will not have that for Katie. I can't fall for a guy who can only give half of himself.'

'And are you, Nadia? Falling for me?' His eyes burned into hers. 'Is that so bad?'

Yes. Yes, it was.

'You make me feel things I haven't felt for a very long time.' Maybe never, she thought. 'It's taken me all this time to rebuild my life. I'm happy with that status quo. Secure in what I have and what I am.'

He put up his hand. 'You're your own woman. I know that. See that.'

'And Katie and I are happy.'

He leaned forward. 'What if I could make you happier? Both of you. A bigger world.'

She heard the words. Wonderful words. But… did she really want that?

'I tried that. I wasn't happier with Alex. And Katie is my first priority now.'

He shook his head. 'For goodness' sake, just because your husband was less than you expected doesn't mean Katie shouldn't have a dad.'

'You don't know anything about Alex.' She glared at him, not wanting this conversation to go there. But she'd been the one who had brought up her marriage.

'No, I don't know anything.' For the first time she detected a glimmer of bitterness in Henry's quiet voice. 'And I really, really would like to. But you're as prickly as a pear.'

She had caused this trap herself. She tried to divert him. 'Pears aren't prickly.'

'Prickly pears are. You're one of those.'

She shifted until their hips weren't touching. 'Nobody asked you to come and pick the fruit with spikes.'

'I know.' He touched her cheek very, very gently and, despite the bitter little spat they'd almost had, she really, really wanted to cover his fingers and hold him there. Feel his warmth and tenderness against her face.

This whole disaster was so stupid and she'd promised herself she would not confuse lust and love again. If she could just keep it to lust.

He went on softly, as if to himself, almost rhyming, 'I have a thing for this particular prickly pear. And no matter what, I cannot change it there.'

'And I don't want to fall for a doctor.' The words fell like stones between them. Silence followed.

When he didn't say anything, she said, 'Can't we just be friends?' Whispered, 'Maybe even friends with benefits, when Katie's not here. Let's not talk about this future stuff. Just enjoy each other's company?'

She watched him as he stopped what he'd been going to say, saw a strange…could it have been hurt, cross his face?

Decisively, he shook his head. 'No. I don't think so.'

'Why not?' And that hadn't sounded like a petulant child. Much.

'Because,' he said simply, with just a little bite,

'a fling is not what I have in mind.' He got up and, to her chagrin, he left.

She wondered if she still had a date.

CHAPTER EIGHTEEN

Henry

HENRY SHUT THE door behind him quietly, careful not to wake Katie, when in fact he wanted to slam it. Friends with benefits. No strings. No commitment.

That way disaster lay—for him, anyway. He didn't want to give up on Nadia—he was falling deeply for her, but equally he couldn't give up being the sort of doctor who was there for his patients. Maybe this wasn't going to work.

He hadn't made it to the lift before his phone vibrated in his pocket. It was a message from his registrar, Amelia. Little Gregory—his heartrate had spiked. He probably should have spent the last couple of hours getting in a power nap because he suspected he'd be up all night.

He chose the down button instead of up and sped out of the door and towards the hospital, lifting his phone as he walked. He stabbed the number for his registrar. 'What's happening, Amelia?'

'Henry, Gregory's temperature just hit forty,' she said, concern clear in her voice. 'I thought you'd want to know.'

'Yes. Always. I'll be there in three minutes.'

'That's good.'

'Is his mother there?'

'Yes.'

'Okay, I'm coming.'

Henry was right. He was up most of the night, but in the early hours of Monday morning Gregory's condition turned the corner and the child settled into a more peaceful sleep.

Henry went home to catch a few hours' rest. When he checked in when he woke, his patient had continued to improve.

Henry felt like a deflated punching bag and decided a run with Malachi might just get him through the day.

Malachi was jogging on the spot when Henry arrived. *Oops.*

'Sorry. Took me a little longer to get here than I thought it would.'

'I'm not that far ahead of you.' Malachi cast him a glance. 'Rough night?'

'You could say that.'

They jogged along, slowly increasing speed. 'I get tricky mums and babies. You get tricky kids.'

It had been a big week with his sick patients, Jake and Gregory. Silence.

Malachi concluded, 'We love what we do.'

Shame everyone didn't, Henry mused silently, thinking of Nadia.

'Does Lisandra love what you do?'

Malachi's expression didn't change. 'She's a midwife. She gets it.'

'And Bella's a nurse, so she gets Simon's work.'

'Which would be Simon's business.' They jogged across a road to a park and began to circle it. Finally, Malachi said, 'You're wondering because Nadia isn't a nurse?'

'I guess.'

His friend grunted. 'She works in the kids' ward. She'll get it.' They ran a few more metres before he added, 'If she loves you enough.'

Henry winced as he ran. And that was the kicker. How did he make that happen? Could he? Of course not. She had to do that.

But Malachi wasn't finished. 'The job isn't worth losing them. The job has to give too. Not just them giving. Learned that.' He didn't speak again while Henry ruminated over the wisdom.

Afterwards, when the burn and aches were showered away, Henry felt the exercise had brought him some calm because, strangely, the slap of their feet on the concrete, the peripheral waves and the cool breeze before the sun came too high and too hot had made him human again.

And those brief words of Malachi's had

smoothed the jagged edges in his brain and strengthened his determination.

He could make this work. He didn't want a benefits-only relationship with Nadia, but at least she wanted that. Or perhaps he wasn't one hundred percent sure that was what Nadia really wanted either.

She'd said she was scared. And she was certainly determined that Katie wouldn't have the childhood disappointments she'd had. He got that. But she wanted a date. She wanted to go out with him. Even a tumble in bed, which just ticked him off because he wasn't a one-night stand kind of man. But maybe he could win by stealth.

For Nadia. For him. For Katie.

By the end of Monday, the antibiotics had kicked in well enough for Lulu's Jake to improve markedly and seeing the tears of relief run down Lulu's face made Henry's own chest ache with relief as well.

Henry slipped an arm around her shoulders and hugged her. Tough being a mum.

'His condition's improved so much we could move him down to the children's ward if you're happy with that, Lulu.'

Lulu nodded. Henry knew she'd felt intimidated by the high-tech drama of the critically ill patients and their beeping, noisy machines that monitored them. And resting more easily would be better for the child than the drama that happened up here. The staff were great in either place. Yes, he could move.

CHAPTER NINETEEN

Nadia

FROM BEHIND THE desk near the door, Nadia watched as Jake was wheeled into the ward in a wheelchair with Lulu hovering behind. A nurse escorted the pale, drowsy boy with his intravenous fluids and the orderly pushing the chair headed for the nurses' station, looking straight ahead. Lulu kept glancing behind, and Nadia saw her face relax when she found Henry had caught up.

Nadia waved at Jake as he passed but the boy's eyes were dull and fixed on his hands, though Lulu smiled at her briefly before snapping back to her son as if she couldn't allow him out of her sight.

Nadia jumped up and hugged her, and then Tara Taylor was up and moving towards them, taking the notes from the nurse and directing the orderly to the room nearest the nurses' station. Nadia went back to her desk. They didn't need a ward clerk in their way.

Oh, poor Lulu. Her hovering fear that her son would be snatched from her still clung and clouded her worried eyes and Nadia felt her heart go out to her. Imagine if that was Katie?

The ensuing efficient organising had Jake in the bed, his IVs sorted and his mother seated in a comfortable chair beside him in minutes. A folded bed was tucked away in the corner for her in the night.

Lulu looked as if she could possibly allow herself to almost relax for the first time in a long time, and Nadia thought about that nursing degree she'd considered taking on, which she'd first considered years ago to attract her father's approval in her teens. Maybe when Katie went to school next year.

Then she thought about the shift work, and the time away from her daughter, and the missing out Katie would suffer without her mother home. Or maybe she didn't need to prove anything any more and could just read about what she wanted to know. No. This was good.

But there was no reason she couldn't study from home and learn more. She had a good brain. It had nothing to do with the fact she wanted to be able to understand Henry's work more. Not that. She knew enough now to know that Jake did look like a sick little boy. The sight made Nadia want to run to the preschool and check that her own Katie was fine.

She suspected strongly that worry about Jake had been an extra stress, along with the immunosuppressed young boy who had worried Henry so much. Being Henry, he would have worried about them both.

Which was probably why, when he appeared at her desk, his skin was pale except for the dark circles under his eyes.

Oh, Henry. She wanted to touch his face but she kept her hands firmly on the desk.

'You look as if you haven't slept since I saw you last.'

'Got a couple of hours.' He smiled at her as if she was as good as a tonic. 'How's Katie?'

'Good.' She waved him on. 'I'm glad Lulu has you looking after Jake.'

Henry smiled. He leaned down and said quietly, 'Are we still on for our date? Friends with benefits even, if that is what you want?'

Nadia blinked with the unexpected reversal. He'd said no. Now it was okay? She didn't understand why she suddenly felt disappointed until she told herself this was a good thing.

She nodded, her cheeks pink. Not meeting his eyes.

'Wednesday. I'll pick you up at six,' he mouthed, and moved away and her gaze followed him. Stuck on his broad back. Silly to be miffed he'd decided just sex was okay. Especially when it had been her idea.

Across the room, Henry touched Lulu's shoulder and the woman turned to him with relief.

She couldn't begrudge Lulu his attention. He was there when her friend needed him the most. She thought that if something like that happened to Katie, how much she'd need to rely on someone like Henry to save her daughter.

How she already had when Katie was born. The thought gave her chills and warred with the promise to never fall for a doctor, which she'd made to herself after years of her father's neglect.

A promise that seemed a little immature and rash now, as an adult. She could feel the wall she'd built crack a little and sag. Reminded herself, *Just friends.* She had a date and she wasn't backing out. She was definitely interested in exploring those benefits…with him.

But Henry's work was important too, he was amazing at what he did, and maybe her dad was too. Imagine that.

She didn't see Henry on Tuesday because the admin clerk in the emergency department had been called home to her sick mother and Nadia had been asked if she could go across and take on that more intense job for the day.

It had been a challenge, learning new procedures, the actual drama and busyness of the emergency ward admissions position compared to her own, but she had finished the long day with a satisfaction that made her wonder just how much she was coasting in the job that she had now.

It also meant she didn't get to see Henry as no paediatric admissions came in, so by the time Wednesday afternoon came she hoped she still had a date that night.

She hadn't heard anything to the contrary, so Katie helped Nadia pack her tiny unicorn suitcase with pyjamas, slippers and dressing gown. Her toothbrush and favourite blanket, plus clothes for the morning, lay on top with Ernestine. Katie didn't sleep over at her great-gran's often, so tonight's sleepover seemed extra exciting.

Nadia felt strange banishing her daughter for a man. For Henry. For sex? Maybe they wouldn't get to third base.

And when it all boiled down Katie would only be downstairs.

When Nadia arrived at Catherine's door, her grandmother shooed her off with an elegant hand. 'Go! Relax, make yourself beautiful. We don't need you here.'

'Well…' she huffed, and escaped the excited Katie much sooner than intended and scurried back down to her unit on the ground floor and fluffed around with a smile on her face.

Good grief, a real date after so many years. Cue leg and armpit shaving, eyebrow plucking, even tooth flossing.

She couldn't quite believe she'd let herself get

to this stage of excitement, but it was only a date. And thank goodness she had previous exposure to Henry over the last couple of weeks or she would have been a mess.

Only Henry. At that thought, she paused. She'd said that before and it hadn't worked then either. Her hand suspended as she mascaraed her lashes.

Just Henry? There was nothing *just* about Henry. Her belly warmed at the thought.

And for a moment, clear as if he were there in the mirror, she could see his mouth. Almost feel his beautiful, beautiful lips on hers. And what that mouth could do. The warmth in her stomach exploded into an inferno and she had to step back and breathe for a moment. Good grief. Where had she been storing those fireworks?

Her chest rose and fell as she tried to shake the all too vivid pictures and just breathe. But she tingled. Tingled?

It didn't mean they would sleep together—it just meant they wouldn't have to constantly be alert for Katie. That was all. Just a date. And she could even dress up. Wins everywhere.

CHAPTER TWENTY

Henry

HENRY KNOCKED ON Nadia's door with one hand and held the bouquet of red roses in the other. Truth be told, his heart did beat just a little faster because he'd pinned a lot of hope on tonight.

One part of him thought the flowers were all too much after they'd already been spending time together, but then his romantic side decided he wanted her to have them. He needed to give them to her.

When Nadia opened the door, her gaze met his with what looked like excitement, thank heaven for that, and relief swamped him.

Then her gaze fell to the flowers. Her eyes went round in surprise.

'Henry? Flowers?' She smiled and the delight he saw made him want to bring her flowers every time he saw her. 'How beautiful. Thank you.'

But she didn't stand aside. She stared at the

flowers while he drank her in, though she still didn't move.

She was as useless as he was, and the indulgent thought calmed him. He asked a question with his hand, and the movement drew her eyes to the door.

She pulled it open. 'Sorry. Come in. You've made me flustered.'

He smiled. Good—surely it was good to be unpredictable? He offered the roses again. 'You take these, I'll shut the door.'

She gathered up the roses. They truly were an armful and the soft dark petals looked so beautiful against her brown skin. 'Thank you, they're glorious.'

She stood there holding them, as if not sure what to do next.

'You put them in water. That way, I don't get stabbed when I kiss you.'

She blinked. And for a horrible moment there he thought he saw tears in her eyes. Maybe the dead husband had brought her flowers along with pain? Had he done the wrong thing?

'I'm sure they would have been de-thorned. Is that a word?'

'Sounds plausible.' He nodded, relieved, at the roses, and she spun and carried them to the kitchen.

He shut the door and followed. Of course. Stood watching by what he was becoming to think of as his wall as she pulled out a big clear vase and filled it with water, his heart full, just drinking her in like the vase drank the water.

When she plonked them instead of taking ages to arrange them, he could not have been more pleased. He slipped up behind her when her hands were free, wrapped his arms around her waist, linking his fingers and thinking suddenly of the popcorn episode.

She spun slowly in his arms, smiling. A gentle sweep of lashes as she lifted her mouth. As he leaned down, he watched her eyes darken and her eyelids flutter closed as he swept her mouth gently back and forth with his, breathing her in, feeling her softness melt under his. He'd needed this. Needed her. Needed her to want him.

When they stepped back both breathed more quickly and, just a little flustered, he murmured, 'You know, I really like your kitchen.'

'Do you?' Her voice husky, not quite steady. Eyes still a little glazed.

He glanced around. More popcorn thoughts. 'In fact, that wall over there looks so promising.'

This time, she focused. Narrowed her eyes. And he laughed.

'Sorry, sorry. Just fantasising. You could try it?' he teased.

She looked at the wall and back at him. Her eyes lingered on his mouth and then ran down the open neck of his button-down shirt and…she had him.

Judging by the gleam in her eyes, she could imagine with the best of them. Henry felt his body heat. Harden.

Her turn to tease him. She smiled. 'We'll have to find out about that later, then. I'll just get my bag,' she said.

Henry had tried to find a restaurant with dancing. He'd even asked a few people, but the looks he'd received hadn't been worth the lack of response.

He'd asked Amelia, thinking his registrar might know. She'd grown up in the Gold Coast. Sure. She'd told him about this fabulous restaurant her mum had told her about, with a real band, and he'd been starting to feel hopeful when she'd said it had closed ten years ago.

Malachi had suggested takeaway with music on at home.

Simon had suggested one of those companies that did picnic hampers, take his own music and dance on the beach.

Who would have thought it would be so hard? In London there'd been plenty of places, but apparently not in the Gold Coast. Instead, he'd decided they'd stick with a local Greek restaurant that they could walk home from. The music would be the sound of the waves. And it was almost a full moon. And on a Wednesday night the yahoos wouldn't be out driving up and down the street in their loud cars.

He watched as she leant to retrieve her purse and he followed the line of her glorious legs to her shoes. High heels. Thinking of footpaths.

'Would you like to walk home? Will your shoes be comfortable for that?'

She turned and smiled at him, nodding. 'Thank you for asking. They should be fine, but I can fit a pair of folding flats in my bag in case.'

He guessed she'd like to walk home too. The idea pleased him.

The restaurant had been painted Mediterranean blue and Santorini white and Malachi had said it was his grandmother's favourite place.

They sat at the bar first and sipped a cocktail called Sex on the Beach. They'd both smiled at that.

When they finished their drink he asked for their secluded table with champagne, and suddenly it was easy.

He told her about London. She told him about the friendships she'd made on the Gold Coast and how she'd found her job. How she'd sometimes thought of a nursing degree, but that would leave Katie being minded too much so maybe she'd wait for a few more years and decide.

He'd always studied and gone where he wanted. A little lost without a family, but not tied down.

'I've never thought about the responsibility of children and their impact on a parent's choice.'

'Especially a single parent.' She sipped the wine, smiling at the taste. 'This is lovely.'

He was still thinking about decisions and choices. 'Is nursing something you've wanted to do for a long time?'

'To be honest, I think I wanted my dad to approve my choice. He always said Isabella should have been a doctor, but she never wanted to be.'

'He never said you should be a doctor?'

'He barely noticed Isabella, and she was the shining light. I was a shadow behind her. He just assumed I'd get married, and I did.'

He took her hand. 'You could never be a shadow.' He shook his head, looking at her in disbelief. 'You blaze every time I see a glimpse of you.' She was so beautiful, vibrant. A force he was drawn to like a lemming to the cliff. Unfortunate simile.

'Thank you.' She smiled at him. 'You are good for my ego, Henry, that's for sure.'

'I'm good for more than that.' He might have said that before.

He watched her expression change in an instant. Eyes and mouth serious. It happened fast. She squeezed his hand back.

'Yes. Of course you are. You're an absolute champion and what you did for Lulu and how you cared for Jake is wonderful. Everyone loves you in the kids' ward and Bella and my grand-mother sing your praises.'

That was a little too much. He tried to squirm away from that line of conversation. Tried to joke. 'And Katie wants to know my favourite pizza.'

'Katie thinks you're wonderful.'

So, he had to ask. 'And you, Nadia. Do you sing my praises?'

'Not enough.' She held his gaze, hers troubled, and he wanted to soothe her fears. 'I'm a bit afraid you want to cosset and keep me safe. Turn me into the little woman. Look after me while you leave me at home.'

Yes. Yes, he did. He saw that now. 'And why does that make you afraid?'

'Our dad was a shadow. But he kept us safe. You couldn't even fight with him because he wasn't there. I like you, a lot, but I don't want a carer. I want a partner. Someone who's there. Or I'll look after myself and Katie.'

'I could do that.' He reached out, caught her fingers in his across the table. Her hand was soft and cool in his.

'Maybe. Maybe not.' Her voice cautiously con-sidering. 'My grandmother thinks Bella and I were scarred by our dad's neglect. I hesitate to say scarred. I'd say wary. He gave us no priority.' She looked up. 'None.'

'You've mentioned that and I hear you.'

'Good.' She nodded. Hearing him hearing her.

'Bella has made it work with Simon, but I think I'm less willing to risk going back to being…accommodating is probably the word…to a profession. Maybe my sister understands more because she's used to shift work as well.'

'You work in a hospital. It's not new for you.' He remembered Malachi's reassurance. If she loved him.

Her eyes explored his as if she wanted to read his thoughts. He wanted to just lose himself there. But she was searching. 'Maybe I'm more selfish? For Katie. I know what I want for her.'

He didn't dispute her right. 'Well, it's hard not to be selfish when you've been responsible for everything for years. It's been up to you to be there for Katie and look after yourself and support yourself.' He shrugged and went on mildly, 'It has been about you surviving. I just happen to think you'd be thriving, not just surviving with me.'

She went to speak but he held up his free fingers. He'd hadn't let her hand get away.

'But I want to nudge in here too. I want to be a part of this.' He waved that free hand to include them both. 'Sit with you on your sofa. Make popcorn. I want to be there to carry Katie to bed at night.'

'Most times she doesn't need carrying.' Nadia frowned.

He brushed that away. 'Have you any idea how

amazing it was, feeling her weight in my arms, her little soft cheek against my neck? Her trust.'

She nodded. 'Yes, I see you genuinely like being with Katie.'

He hoped she knew he'd protect Katie with all his being.

Maybe it was time to share a few truths. She had shared hers. But he hated saying it. 'My father was an alcoholic. He left when I was seven. When I have a family, they will never want for anything. It's a factor in my wanting to succeed. My wife will not work herself to death like my mother did.'

She sat back, pulling her hand free. 'That's why you put your work first,' she said quietly. It was not a question. 'Why you're so dedicated.' She looked more sad than enlightened, and he wished he hadn't said anything now. He had the feeling that somehow that hadn't helped his cause. 'You're a good man.'

'And I agree to going slow. Except for the "benefits", if they're still on the table. I'm not that good a man.'

She whispered, 'I was hoping for something softer than a table.' He felt her gaze slide to his mouth. Even more softly, she said, 'You do kiss like a dream.'

'Tonight?' He tried to recover some of the ground he suspected he'd lost.

'I'll think about that. As for the future, you'd

have to be there, and I can see how a lot of the time you might not be.'

Yes, he might need to work on that.

CHAPTER TWENTY-ONE

Nadia

OVER THE SOFT sounds of the restaurant around them Nadia's phone vibrated in her purse. Sadly, it wasn't a soft buzz like Henry's, it was a noisy one.

He sat back and she pulled it out. 'Excuse me.' Frowned at it. 'It's Bella. She knows we're out. I have to phone her back.'

'Of course.' Henry picked up his menu. 'I'll decide what to eat.'

She heard him but she wasn't listening. She was walking away from the table, waiting for the phone to answer. 'Bella, are you okay? Is it Gran or Katie?'

There was silence for too long and Nadia's heart-rate picked up. Then her sister said very softly, 'Gran and Katie are fine. I need you to come to me.' The sentence was short and breathless. 'Take me to the hospital.'

'Yes, of course. Where's Simon?'

Several deep breaths later she said, 'They're doing an exchange transfusion. On a baby. And I know he can't leave.'

'Labour? You're in labour?' Had to be.

A puff of breath into the phone. Could have been an unamused laugh. 'Yes.'

'We're on our way.' She glanced at Henry and remembered that they didn't have a car. Uber, then. Bella had a car and if they got to her, they could use hers.

'Less than five minutes. We'll be there.'

'Hurry.'

'Bella?' This sounded very unlike her calm sister. 'Maybe you should get that ambulance as well.'

'Kai's just gone to sleep. If I wake him, he'll scream and I can't do that right now.'

'We're coming. Phone the ambulance anyway.' She clicked off and spun back to Henry, who had stood. Of course he'd read her distress and was ready to go. 'Something's wrong with Bella. She said labour, but maybe more.'

She reached for her bag, which Henry had picked up as she came back to the table. 'Can you call an Uber and get us there? She's got a car we can use. I've told her to call an ambulance, but for some reason she doesn't want to.'

He nodded. Handed the concerned waiter fifty dollars and waved him away. Scanned his apps and typed for the ride, saying as an aside, 'Where's Simon?'

'Something about an exchange transfusion. At the hospital.'

The Uber pulled up as they descended the escalator from the restaurant to the street. She saw Henry glance at his phone and then the number-plate on the car before opening her door to usher her in.

When they arrived at Bella's front door six minutes later, it was open but Bella wasn't there. Heeding her sister's request that Kai should not be woken, she called out quietly, 'Bella?'

'In the lounge,' she heard.

When they entered the room Bella wasn't resting quietly in a chair or on the lounge, where Nadia expected her to be.

Her sister was on the floor and for a moment she thought she'd fallen, lying half on her side and half on her back and packed with cushions from the settee. There was even a cushion under her bottom. Bella's feet were up on the coffee table.

Henry took one look at her and knelt down beside her. 'I'm guessing cord prolapse.'

'What?' said Nadia, trying to grasp what he'd understood so quickly.

Bella smiled an unconvincing smile. 'Very good, Henry.' Then her face contorted. 'And now I want to push.'

Henry frowned. 'Any chance of waiting for an ambulance?'

'No,' she panted and pushed. When the contraction was past, she licked dry lips and whispered, 'It would be all lights and sirens and awkward positioning and people who don't really have a lot of experience like you and I about this. This way, I have some control. Different if I felt there was time for a Caesarean before the birth.'

'I don't know what I'm doing,' said Nadia softly, but she was talking to Henry.

'I do,' said Bella. 'And Henry does.'

Some of the horror and the pressure of helplessness left. She was right, Henry was here. Since everyone else was ridiculously calm, then she'd better follow suit.

'Since you're busy, Henry had better tell me what he wants me to do.'

'You could find some towels. Turn on the heaters, Nadia. Warm the room up even more for the baby. Maybe pass your sister a drink of water.'

He touched Bella's shoulder, and she opened her eyes from where she'd been breathing quietly in some calming place in her mind. 'Do you have an ultrasound Doppler to listen to the baby's heartrate? I know what you midwives are like. You've always got one tucked away in a cupboard.'

Bella laughed very, very softly, part groan. 'I do. It's on the dressing table in my room.'

Nadia felt his glance and she stood. Something else she could do, she thought as she hurried from the room. She heard him saying, 'Have you told Simon anything?'

'I tried, but I couldn't speak to the ward nurse.' She sniffed. 'I was afraid I'd just cry all over the phone and then he'd rush and not think. So I rang Nadia.'

Henry nodded. 'Good plan, we've got you covered. I'm just going to make a quick call…' His voice faded as Nadia ran into Bella and Simon's room and grabbed the little baby listener off the dressing table.

By the time she was back, Henry had called through to Simon. She heard him say, 'Bella's in labour. She says it's imminent. Cord prolapse. Couldn't talk to tell you.' He held the phone away from his ear. 'I'll see you soon, then.' And smiled down at Simon's wife. He whispered, 'I think you're in trouble.'

'No time,' she gasped. 'I'm pushing.'

Nadia handed Henry the foetal ultrasound machine. She'd found a bottle of gel too, remembering the midwives had always put it on the end before they'd listened when she'd been pregnant with Katie.

Henry pressed to the spot Bella suggested.

Instantly, they heard the galloping heartbeats, so reminiscent of the hoofbeats of a horse, and

Bella must have decided it was good because she sagged with relief.

'Clever baby,' she whispered, and a tear trickled from the corner of her eye.

Henry sent Nadia a reassuring smile. 'Strong normal rate.'

So they were reassured by the strong beat. Nadia almost believed them, but her gaze was drawn to the loop of thick purple umbilical cord that was hanging between Bella's legs. She knew at least it was wrong to have the cord before the baby.

'Don't we need scissors and cord clamps? For the placenta after?' Nadia felt useless and ill-educated. She should have studied more, but Katie was almost five and she'd forgotten all the things she'd read.

'Lotus birth until it's all over,' Bella said.

Nadia looked at Henry. 'What?'

'If it comes then just leave the placenta attached—wrap it up in a towel still joined to baby and out of the way.'

They were so calm. So in tune. And she was swirling in a whirlpool of fear which she suddenly realised wasn't helping anyone. *Stop it*, she told herself. *Have faith.* She could be calm.

Henry was saying to Bella, 'How was your birth with Kai?'

'Fast.'

'You should do that again,' Henry urged gently.

They heard a car screech to a halt outside and Bella winced. 'There'll be tyre marks on the new driveway.'

Henry bit back a smile. 'I'm guessing now you can push?'

They all glanced towards the pounding footsteps.

And then Simon was in the room, skidding onto his knees towards his wife. 'Good timing,' she breathed and pushed.

As far as Nadia could tell, even then there seemed very little progress, and as if her sister thought so too, Bella muttered, 'It's because I'm lying like this. I can't push uphill.'

'What about the pressure on the cord?' Simon spoke quietly, but with no dispute in his voice.

Bella huffed. 'Did you see the cord? It's like an anchor rope. All that fat jelly should protect for the time it will take.'

'Then move where you want to, my love, and let's see our child.' He helped her up.

As soon as Bella was kneeling on towels in front of the coffee table with her elbows resting on the table and holding Simon's hand, things started to happen.

Simon waved with his hand. 'Make a little bed for Bella, Nadia, next to her here, so she can slide down with the baby on her skin afterwards.'

Nadia gathered a few towels and a cushion and brought the blanket over ready.

Henry was down the business end and Nadia slipped a few more folded towels beside him and marvelled at everyone else's composure.

Simon and Bella were concentrating together, as if Simon could will strength and power into his wife.

Henry knelt like a statue, a calm statue, holding an open towel and waiting. He said softly, 'We need the exact time, Nadia, Your job. Then tell me when it's thirty seconds after birth.'

Nadia nodded and moved behind him, tears running down her cheeks, a hand on his shoulder. That was all she could do to help her sister, and watch the medical people in the room save a life. 'I can do that.'

And then Henry was saying, 'Coming now, Bella, nice and smooth…' And then, 'Head's out…' And her sister heaved a sigh.

'We won't stop for this one, Bella—keep going,' Henry murmured, and Bella pushed on.

'Perfect, one shoulder and now the other.' There was a flurry of movement and shiny, tiny limbs, a splash of fluids and more cord and suddenly the baby was there.

Nadia's heart leapt at the pale child who hadn't been there a second ago and now lay unmoving in Henry's hands.

Mindful of her one job, Nadia glanced at the clock. It was a big clock, with hands and a second hand, and she said, 'Three minutes and fifteen seconds past eight.'

Then Henry was rubbing, murmuring, 'A girl. Stunned. She's not breathing, but still has tone, heartrate around eighty. So, looking good.'

She didn't look good to Nadia, but Henry was smiling as he dried the baby and put his hand again on the chest. 'Heartrate one hundred. Grimacing like crazy. Come on, baby—a big breath. You know you can do it.'

'Ivy. Her name is Ivy. Come on, Ivy...' Now Bella wept, and Simon was rubbing her neck and shoulders, soothing, telling her she was wonderful, that baby would be fine and Henry had this.

Just as Nadia called, 'Thirty seconds,' with her chest tight—oh, heavens, when would this baby cry?—Ivy sucked in a shuddering breath, coughed, squeaked and then roared with disapproval at her rapid arrival.

Nadia burst into tears, Bella pulled off her nightie to bare her skin and, trailing the ridiculously long cord, she shifted from where she knelt to the bed Nadia had made, making give-to-me motions with her hands as she lay down.

Henry handed the baby to Simon, who placed her against her mother's skin as Bella's hands wrapped around her newborn. Simon covered them both with a towel and a blanket, tucking them in and leaving just a tiny face turned sideways against her mother's bare skin. Wailing complaints kept coming from under the blanket. The little face had already turned pink.

Finally, Ivy settled and snuffled. Henry whispered to Nadia, 'Skin to skin against the mother. Fastest way to settle heartrate and breathing and keep a baby warm.'

'Oh.' She hadn't known that. But Henry had. And Bella and Simon. Yes, she'd start reading about midwifery and paediatrics.

Simon was stroking Bella's hair, his face aglow with the release of tension, replaced with joy. 'You always wanted a home birth,' he teased his wife as he kissed her cheek, such relief in his voice.

Bella's shoulders dropped and she breathed out a huge sigh. 'There's something to be said for all the medical equipment, my love, in emergencies. We'll go into Maternity next time.'

Nadia blinked. 'Next time?'

Henry laughed and once the afterbirth had arrived, he wrapped it and placed it beside Bella at the end of the impossibly long cord until they could sever the connection. Simon wanted samples of the oxygen and carbon dioxide levels in the umbilical cord. Even if delayed, he thought they could get them, so the men were sorting the logistics of that.

Fifteen minutes later, Nadia helped Bella shower while the men examined Ivy and pronounced her well. A midwife had arrived to sort the cord gases and Bella would be transferred soon.

Simon wanted Bella to stay one night in the hospital to rest, so the staff could watch Ivy, but still Nadia had been surprised when her sister had agreed.

'Just to keep an eye on Ivy overnight,' Bella said, 'then I'm home.'

And soon they were gone, leaving Nadia and Henry at the door.

'I was terrified,' Nadia said as they watched Simon's car pull away from the house.

'Me too,' Henry agreed.

'Oh, you were not.' Nadia pushed his arm and he smiled. 'You were as cool as a cucumber. So was Bella.'

He tucked her back into his side as they closed the door. 'You held it together well too, you know. Because we all knew that panic was more dangerous than anything else.'

Good grief. Had they really been terrified like her? Now, that was scary.

Henry went on, 'And there are protocol steps to follow for just such occasions.'

'Even when you're not an obstetrician? Paediatricians don't have cord prolapses.'

He laughed. 'Proved that wrong tonight. But we have the training in it. Still, I've seen my share, and the treatment is rapid Caesarean section. And keeping pressure off the cord until you can get to a hospital.'

'But Ivy is okay?'

'Still very lucky. But Bella had pressure, knew it was imminent. Even though the baby's hard skull crushes the cord against the bony pelvis and occludes the blood supply during birth.'

'So no oxygen gets through?'

'Some does, but less than needed, more often. The fatter the cord with the jelly, the more chance the baby has of the blood vessels inside the cord not becoming too compressed, letting good oxygen flow through.'

'Sounds risky.'

'In an imminent birth like Bella's, sometimes it's faster to push the baby out, despite cord compression. That's less desirable if it was a first baby, which could be slow. Which is why I asked Bella how her first labour went.'

Nadia remembered. 'She said fast.'

He nodded, blowing out a breath. 'Never so glad to hear something.'

Nadia nodded. 'And you said, "You should do that again".'

'Yes. Push baby out now, was what I was saying.' He smiled. 'Having such a thick cord was a big bonus. And probably why the heartrate we listened to, before the birth, was so perfect. Baby wasn't affected, despite the way the cord had been exposed to air, which makes it contract.'

She couldn't hear enough about the mechanics of this, though Henry was looking at her as if to say, *Surely that's all you want to hear?*

'Last question. So you're saying, the thicker the cord, the more Wharton's jelly protecting the blood vessels means blood supply and oxygen from the placenta. And that's why Bella had her feet up on the table when we arrived.'

'Yes. Gravity to keep the baby's head from pressing on the cord until help arrived.'

'And Bella knew that?'

'Yes, she's a midwife. It's protocol. But the situation was dangerous for baby.'

Nadia shook her head. Her sister. 'She looked so calm. Even when the baby didn't breathe.' Nadia's remembered dread hit her. Delayed reaction. Tears flooded her eyes again. She would never forget her pale and limp little niece.

Henry put his arm around her shoulders. 'Ivy had lots of tone. And reflexes. Heartrate was there, if not fast. As long as there's a heartbeat, most babies will pull back and revive well.'

Maybe she didn't want to be a doctor or a nurse, with all this responsibility. She liked being a photographer.

He squeezed her shoulders. 'Ivy's had a feed, which is what she needed after the stress of the birth. Like Katie, Ivy's a fighter.'

Nadia slipped her arm around his waist, the

man was rock-solid, and he squeezed back. She did feel better just hearing that.

In fact, she really did have so much history with this man, even though Henry had only been back in Australia a few weeks. Between them there was Katie's history. Now Ivy's. All of it with Henry being there for her.

She looked up at him. 'All I know is I'm very glad you were here, Henry. And glad Bella was the mother who knew what she was doing.'

Henry laughed quietly. 'That she did. And with Simon arriving we had plenty of neonatal backup.'

CHAPTER TWENTY-TWO

Henry

HENRY SAVOURED THE feel of Nadia's arm around his waist. This was what he wanted. A family home like this. And Nadia to relax with after a tense medical situation.

She'd done well as a non-medical person. She hadn't panicked. She'd been quick and helpful, almost like a scout nurse in Theatre.

He smiled at the thought. He guessed she'd seen drama in the children's ward at times and that might have prepared her. Or the fact she came from medical people.

Sadly, their date had come to an end, but he wouldn't have it any other way with such a great outcome for Bella and Simon.

'How about we order takeaway while we wait for Simon to come home?'

'Sounds good. Bella didn't seem to think that Kai would wake so we can make ourselves comfortable.'

He eyed Simon's big comfy sofa. Nice idea that. 'What would you like to eat? I'm happy to ring the restaurant. I'm pretty sure they'll allow Uber Eats to pick up a Greek meal. Especially if we promise to make another booking next week.'

Nadia leaned her head against him as if thinking. 'Why don't we go back next week and try again? And order some pasta tonight. I know that Simon likes his red wine. There's bound to be half a dozen bottles of nice Shiraz in the wine rack.'

Henry grinned. 'You don't think he'll be upset if we drink his best wine?'

She giggled. He loved that sound. It was rare and lovely and he breathed her in, savouring their closeness. And there was closeness after what they'd shared tonight.

'We won't take the Shiraz he's saving for a special occasion.' She laughed. 'We'll order some pasta for Simon as well. That will cheer him up when he comes home.'

Nadia went in and checked on Kai for the second time and Henry wondered if she was missing Katie or just nervous after all the excitement.

She'd told him her grandmother had texted and said that she and Katie had had a lovely evening and now Katie and Ernestine were asleep. Nadia had texted back and told her the news and the good outcome.

As Henry searched for the number, he smiled at the inclusion the doll had in the adults' conversations. He wasn't ordering food for Ernestine, but he did like that sweet indulgence of a little girl's fantasies.

And he had Nadia to himself tonight as soon as Simon arrived. Hopefully, not too far away. The back door opened, no noisy tyre-screech this time, and Simon walked in.

He came straight to Henry and clapped him on the back. 'Thanks, Henry. For looking after Bella and Ivy. I owe you.'

'You looked after Katie and Nadia.' He grinned. 'We're square. And congratulations on your new dramatic daughter.'

Simon laughed, his voice still tinged with relief. 'Hopefully not an indication of things to come with Ivy.' He glanced up at the sky. 'Please heaven.'

He acknowledged Nadia as she came from Kai's room. 'Hey, Nadia. He's asleep?'

'Yes. Out for the count.'

'Thank you. We certainly intruded on your date night.'

She smiled, waved it away, and Henry said, 'That's okay.' He gestured to Nadia. 'Your sister-in-law suggested we borrow one of your many red wines and take it away with us when the pasta arrives.'

Simon looked hopeful. 'Pasta? There's pasta?'

'Coming. Your dinner. And ours,' Nadia said with a smile, and turned for the door when the doorbell rang.

They stayed another twenty minutes, eating with Simon, after phone calls to Gran and Nadia's father—who, strangely, hadn't asked to speak to Nadia, which Henry felt offended by—they could both see Simon needed the company for a little longer.

Eventually, his friend looked more relaxed and waved them away. Clutching their wine, they left in the Uber that arrived to transport them back to the apartments.

Henry opened the door and stood back. Nadia hadn't been to his apartment since he'd moved in and he hoped she liked it.

He watched her face as he pushed open the door and, judging by the way her eyes opened wide and she looked back at him with delight, it did meet with her approval.

Doubt was banished as she breathed, 'Oh, Henry, it's lovely. Did you put this together yourself?'

His pleasure brought a smile. 'I was going for the Hampton look. White and blue, because that's what's outside, with some sandy accents like the beach below.'

'It certainly works. I feel relaxed just looking

at the furnishings and yet it's very different to Bella's decorating.'

He remembered the first time he'd seen Nadia in here and the crowd who had wonderfully forced them onto the veranda to talk. He wasn't looking to have big social events, just wanted Nadia and Katie to feel as if they could come here any time they wanted.

Because he wanted them here all the time and he wanted it nice for them. He hadn't realised that before.

'Yes. But I took your advice and Elsa Green from downstairs, your grandmother's friend, has a cleaner who comes up and waters my plants. She housekeeps and puts the slow cooker on twice a week, so I have proper meals.'

'Lucky you,' she said, but she looked pleased he'd listened.

He'd done it for her and Katie. Wanted it perfect, and things could get messy when he was called out often.

'I know. I can't predict which delicious smells will hit me when I walk in the door on Mondays and Wednesdays.'

She sat down, leaving a space for him on the end of the couch. 'That's good. I was worried about you eating enough. I think you've lost weight since you arrived.'

She worried about him? A good start to tonight.

'It's probably loss of muscle because I haven't had time to go to the gym as often as I did in London.'

She pretended to assess him. 'Nope. None missing. Though you do spend a lot of time lazing around, eating popcorn and drinking wine,' she teased.

But, underneath the banter, something shimmered between them, and he carried the bottle she'd cadged off her brother-in-law and put it on the low table in front of her.

'Don't blame me for that. You're the one encouraging me with bad habits.'

Then he crossed back to the kitchen for the glasses on the counter, along with the candles and matches.

He'd hoped they'd come back here, hence the preparation, and lit the candles so he could turn the lights down.

On the way to the sofa, he slid open the veranda door to allow in the breeze, and the sounds of the ocean that followed it, and set down the glasses. 'Do you still fancy wine?'

'Sure.' She patted her flat stomach. 'I don't need anything more to eat, though.'

He smiled. The pasta had been filling. 'We can have tea or coffee if you'd prefer.'

She laughed. 'No, I'd love another glass of that lovely Margaret River red. Simon really does have great taste.'

He stood for a moment, just to soak her in, sitting on his couch, before he lowered himself beside her.

She was watching him, not the wine, and he leaned in and kissed her gently. 'I've been waiting to do that all night.'

'Mm-hmm, she said and kissed him back. Not gently.

They never did have more wine.

CHAPTER TWENTY-THREE

Nadia

NADIA WOKE AT one a.m. as Henry slipped from the bed. He pressed the blankets around her and kissed her forehead. She suffered only a little embarrassed heat when she considered how he'd drawn such an enthusiastic, and loud, response from her. Several times. More than several.

'Snuggle in. I'll be back.'

He dressed quickly. Leaving? But the bed was warm, her limbs felt like simmering syrup, so she closed her eyes though her smile had dimmed. After what they'd shared, Henry was leaving. Hospital. Couldn't they have their first night without his work interrupting?

But she couldn't stay awake after the unexpected delights Henry had gifted her with and drifted back to sleep.

The next time she woke he was sliding in beside her, his skin cool and his muscular body hard, and deliciously masculine. He was back. Still half asleep, she rolled into him, pulling him closer, slipping her arms around his neck and lifting her face for his kiss.

Henry didn't need a second invitation and by the time they dropped off to sleep that time it was almost dawn.

She woke with Henry's arms around her, his gentle hands cupping her breasts and his body spooning her back, his warm breath on her neck.

Inside, a part of her revelled in the wantonness and the delight of being here, naked with this amazing man whose company she'd come to enjoy so much, and another part panicked at how much she wanted him, loved being with him, and that he'd left her already once. She'd rushed into a step she should have slowed for.

Why couldn't she banish those ridiculous fears that this wouldn't work? So many reasons why it should. Yet a tiny panic built in her belly, though she tried to push it down.

'This is a dream come true, you know.' Henry's deep purring rumble made gooseflesh prickle her skin.

She hadn't realised he was awake and rolled onto her back so she could see his face. His hands slid away and instantly she wanted them back. 'What dream was that?'

'The one where I get called to work then come

back and you put your arms around me and warm me so much we burn the sheets.'

He dreamed of being called to work?

'You leaving the bed seems a bit of a nightmare to me.'

He pulled her close against him and kissed her. 'Best kind of nightmare, climbing back in, though.'

She tensed. Cleared her throat. 'Not my dream.'

She could tell he was still in sexy land when he asked, 'What's your dream?'

'You missed the point.' Her frown deepened. 'I'm pretty sure it would be better if you didn't have a job that dragged you out of bed in the middle of the night.' And the middle of the weekend. And the middle of a lunch. But she didn't add that. With some difficulty.

'All part of the game.' Henry was moving on. 'But, dearest Nadia, it was a wonderful date night.' His voice deepened. 'And morning.'

She wasn't sure she'd moved on. But her skin heated just with that look and he dragged her along.

'Action-packed.' She tried for nonchalance despite her erratic thoughts, half annoyed, half drunk with his obvious appreciation.

'Complete with champagne, emergency birth and our bed.'

Our bed? The thought shocked her. Stupidly, she blurted, 'Your bed. Not mine. Not ours.'

'Ours. It will be here waiting for you.' He kissed her again as if he couldn't resist and slipped from *their* bed.

Yet, despite all the ups and downs of her see-saw thoughts, he was magnificent. Magnetic. But shadows lay beneath his eyes, a man who had been out in the night, many nights, and suddenly she thought of Lulu despite her own stupid angst.

'Henry?'

He turned back.

'Is Jake okay? It wasn't him that called you out, was it?'

He smiled. 'No, Jake's fine. Thank you for asking. He'll probably go home on Friday.'

'Oh.' Now she felt out of line. But her father wouldn't have answered her. 'Okay. I'm glad. Thank you.'

'Thank you,' he said, and she wasn't sure what he was thanking her for.

Once the bathroom door shut, she put her head back on the pillows and stared at the ceiling. What had she done? What had she promised by coming here? Staying. Giving herself like she'd never done before. She remembered Henry's 'our bed'.

They'd resolved nothing. Just made everything more complicated. But she'd done nothing wrong. They were both single. Nothing irretrievable. Surely.

Of course it felt awkward, but not too awkward for a first morning after a night before. And she had discovered Henry Oliver had hidden talents because, no doubt at all, she'd never felt so satisfied and sated, ever. Or was that because she'd felt as if they'd connected on a deeper level than she'd planned for. No. It wasn't that. Please.

Because she still did have doubts that she could be happy with Henry as the man in her life. A part-time man.

She rolled from the sheets, picked up her clothes, dressed and made the bed. Finally, she smoothed the pillows and straightened the quilt—wanting, for some bizarre reason, to erase her visit? No, not erase, but make his room look as immaculate as it had last night when they'd come in.

Her mind flicked back to that moment. Not that she'd had much time to notice in the rush they'd both been in to lose their clothes. He made her feel so hot.

For goodness' sake. She was all over the place.

She wanted her own apartment, and she wanted to be there when Gran called to say Katie was ready to come home, but she couldn't just slip away. Could she?

She went through to the kitchen and put the jug on for Henry to have coffee. On the corner bench she found the latest espresso maker, not what she wanted to figure out now, but she switched it on as well, just in case he wanted to use it.

Henry arrived with little delay, hair still damp

and a bead of moisture in the diamond of his throat, and her doubts morphed into a need so unexpected, so overwhelming she gripped the counter with her hands.

His shirt hung unbuttoned, broad, damp chest beneath, with his tie ready to be knotted as it draped around his collar. This morning there were dancing giraffes on the pattern, but it was the brown expanse of skin that held her gaze. Ripples of wide muscled chest.

The need to lick that tiny droplet on his neck slammed into her, and the wanting to slide against him all over again made her treacherous fingers tighten on the bench behind her.

'If you keep looking at me like that, I'm going to be late for work.' The deep timbre of his voice raised the hairs on her arms. Who was she? What had he done to her last night?

She licked dry lips and conjured up her lost voice, which seemed to have lodged somewhere in her throat. 'I'm ready to go. Get organised downstairs.' She waved a distracted hand at the kitchen. 'I didn't know whether you wanted me to make you some breakfast.'

He crossed the room to her, and she couldn't have stopped her hands sliding under the flaps of that open shirt. His skin felt warm and deliciously damp. And so well-packed. Her face leaned of its own volition into his neck and her tongue licked the water bead that had caught her eye.

He sucked in a breath and the flesh under her hands went rigid. Lost again in a power she hadn't known she possessed, she smiled as she ran her palms around his muscle-covered ribs, couldn't have stopped herself if she'd been threatened with death. His skin felt just as hot and smooth and delicious as she'd known it would.

He groaned. 'We need to talk.'

They did and she knew she wasn't being fair.

'Talk? You mean about the fact we couldn't have one night without you being called away?'

'Not that. Not now.' He leaned down and nipped her lip. 'We're gonna do this again, aren't we? You're not going to disappear again behind the shield?'

Her watch chimed and she thought of Katie, who was probably awake now. She blinked. What was she doing? Who was this woman? She stepped back. 'I'm going for a shower.' She turned for the door, but he caught her arm.

'One more kiss,' he murmured as his arms came around her, his turn to slide fingers on skin, and very, very gently and slowly he made her forget the world.

Before she left, he said, 'And we won't always ask your grandmother to mind Katie. She can always come over too.'

So then she and Katie could both wait until he came back to them from wherever he was called away to?

CHAPTER TWENTY-FOUR

Nadia

HENRY PHONED AT LUNCHTIME. 'Have you chosen a place for lunch?'

'I only just said goodbye to you this morning.' *And my head is still whirling*, she thought, but didn't say because her heartrate had jumped at the sound of his voice.

'It's Thursday,' he said, as if that explained everything.

She didn't answer so he added, 'I like interrupting your work to make sure you eat.'

She smiled at that. Couldn't help it. She'd been smiling and scowling all morning, along with the swings of Will-I-won't-I?

'Well, I've lots of food here. Why don't you just come to my place? I'll whip something up.'

'Perfect. Never too early for bondage,' his voice low and liquid.

She spluttered into the phone. 'I hope you didn't say that from the children's ward.'

'I'll see you at twelve-thirty.' She could hear the smile in his voice, and she suspected he could be taking a little revenge for her comments in the kitchen this morning.

She made a quiche Lorraine and salad. Heated a couple of tiny dinner rolls and set it all out on her patio, humming. Her apartment overlooked the complex garden, behind a low wall. She could see through the foliage but people couldn't see in. Maintaining it was not her responsibility, thankfully, but definitely her pleasure, especially when the walled and paved courtyard gave an extra space for her, with a tiny table and chairs. She'd even put the umbrella up.

By twelve-forty-five she wondered if this was going to work.

The text came in at one p.m.

So sorry, Nadia. Frantic here. But I promise I'll pick up you and Katie to go see the baby at five. I'll be there.

Okay. It was an impromptu lunch. Not a planned one. And he had texted and made a real, promised plan. She picked up one of the still warm bread rolls and nibbled it. And then collected the food to put it all back in the fridge.

They could take the quiche with them to Bella's to see the baby. She'd slipped up to the maternity ward to see Bella earlier. She and Simon would be home by now, and Bella had suggested Nadia could drop in after preschool pick-up.

Henry had been busy at lunchtime. She understood. She did. He was in charge of paediatric emergency admissions and of course there would be children needing him.

She looked at the roll in her hand and suddenly tossed it into the bin. Poured herself a glass of water, drank, and went back to work.

At three o'clock Katie bounced into the car, full of talk of her friends. For the first time all day, Nadia felt like herself as she listened.

Until Katie said, 'Is Dr Henry coming for dinner?'

Was he?

'Maybe. He's coming to take us to Auntie Bella's at five o'clock.'

'In his car? Has he got a little screen for the back of my seat?'

'Yes, in his car. And no to the screen. But Auntie Bella has a big surprise to show you. We're going to visit her.'

'A surprise with Dr Henry?' Almost a happy shout. 'Is Kai there? And Mr Teeny. Is it a present?'

Nadia glanced in the rear-view mirror. Her daughter's eyes were wide with anticipation. 'Yes, Kai will be there. Yes, Mr Tierney too. And no, not a present for you. But we've got one for Auntie Bella.'

After visiting Bella at the hospital, Nadia had slipped into her favourite craft store and found a tiny handmade lemon and green sundress for Ivy. The best was a green headband stitched with tiny leaves.

She considered possible germs from childcare and vulnerable new babies. 'You can have a bath and get changed out of your play clothes and put on one of your pretty dresses.' She hoped they wouldn't have to fight about an early bath.

Katie looked thoughtful. 'I'll put on my princess dress for Dr Henry. He will like that one.'

They'd have to sort that name. Dr Henry wasn't the perfect way for a four-year-old to address her mother's boyfriend. Lover? Maybe partner? She so wasn't sure this was going to work.

By five o'clock they'd both showered and dressed, Katie complete with silver crown, and Nadia had reapplied her make-up.

At ten past five Katie was talking to Ernestine in a cross little voice with much foot stamping.

Five minutes later, the phone rang. 'I'm sorry, Nadia…' Henry's voice. She listened as he ran down his excellent reasons.

'I understand,' she said and then she hung up.

Katie cried, big rolling tears. Suddenly, Nadia had a flashback to a horrible day when her big sister Bella had cried at her tenth birthday. Their father had not made it home for cake and forgotten her birthday dinner.

Something wild and angry and determined, maybe from then, maybe from now, but fury, blossomed in Nadia's chest. *Enough is enough.* She'd known this wouldn't work. He'd hurt Katie. And she shouldn't have believed him enough to tell Katie, so it was her fault too.

'It's okay, sweetheart. We'll ask Gran if she'll come with us.' She should have done that instead anyway. So many things she'd got wrong since she'd left that man's bed this morning.

Was it only this morning?

'You know Gran loves your princess dress very much and Auntie Bella does too. You can show Mr Tierney. I bet he will love it too.' She was gabbling and made herself stop.

Half an hour later they met Gran in the car park. Katie murmured quietly, 'Is it Auntie Bella's birthday?' The exuberance gone.

'It's somebody's birthday.'

'Whose birthday?'

'If I tell you, it won't be a surprise.'

Catherine opened the front passenger door. 'Say hello to Gran.'

'Hello, Gran.'

Her grandmother cast an indulgent glance to the back of the car before she slid in. 'Hello, Katie. Hello, Nadia. Isn't this exciting?'

Katie piped up, a little brighter. 'Mummy said Auntie Bella has a surprise.'

'She certainly has.' Gran laughed. 'Goodness me.' She studied Nadia. 'You've had a big twenty-four hours.'

'Yes.'

'You seem to have lost that glow you had this morning.'

'Really? No, I'm fine.'

'Oh, dear.' Gran shook her head. 'That word. Fine. You sound like your sister.'

She had no idea what Gran was talking about. Or she pretended she didn't.

A quietly excited Mrs Tierney took them through to the sitting room, where Bella looked amazing considering she'd had a precipitous birth the day before and left hospital at lunchtime today.

Baby Ivy lay quietly content and no worse for her rapid and exciting catapult into the world as she nursed at her mother's breast.

Katie's eyes went as wide as frisbees as she stared at the little baby and the almost trim Bella. 'Your baby's out of your tummy, Auntie Bella!' she cried.

The adults laughed. 'Yes, she is, darling. This is Ivy. She's Kai's little sister.'

The aforementioned Kai, head buried under his mother's other arm, was watching the baby with suspicious eyes, but as soon as Simon came back into the room he recovered. Simon had taken leave for the next week to be the bonded parent for his son—and he tickled him until the little boy giggled and recovered his good humour as his daddy swung him on to his shoulder.

'Kai's still getting used to sharing his mummy,' Bella said calmly. 'This is when dads come in handy for diversional therapy.'

'Is that all I'm good for?' Simon pretended to be offended.

'You stack the dishwasher well,' his wife offered, but the loving look which passed between them made Nadia even more aware of what she would not have with Henry. Done deal.

She knew how it felt to have that world ripped away.

Simon took Kai and Katie outside to play on the new capsule trampoline that Mr Tierney and Simon had set up earlier in the week and Mrs Tierney arrived with a pot of tea and three cups.

'Isn't she just beautiful?' Mrs Tierney seemed to glow with her excitement for the new arrival, as Bella sat Ivy up to burp.

Nadia nodded and smiled, and watched her grandmother carry her cup away as the two older ladies drifted from the room to see something in the kitchen.

Gran asked Mrs Tierney about her grandchildren, proving how much a part of this world the Tierneys had become already. It seemed that Bella could let people into her world without expectations. Nadia wondered why she couldn't do that herself.

She looked at her sister. Serene, glowingly happy and so in control. All her life, it had seemed that Bella had a handle on everything. Except for that one birthday. Funny how that had stuck with her today.

Nadia had thought she had control too. Until Henry. She had for a while. Sorting her life after the horror of sudden widowhood and single prembaby parenting, to a settled and secure world after Alex's death.

But since Henry had pushed himself into her life her world had destabilised, and now she didn't feel in control at all. But then, what was control? And how much had she really had anyway? None, apparently.

Bella patted the seat beside her. 'Come sit with me, Nadia.'

Nadia hesitated. She knew Bella had recognised her unhappiness, and was going to grill her. Years of older sister counselling made her aware that she was an open book to Bella. But her sister had enough on her plate without Nadia dumping her stupid concerns and conundrums on her.

Bella patted the seat again. 'Sit. I need to thank you for all your help with Ivy's dramatic arrival yesterday.'

She blinked. Sat. And shook her head. 'I didn't do anything. Henry did it all.'

Bella raised her brows. 'Don't be silly. You did what I had complete faith you'd do. You came. Instantly. As I knew you would. Even when I interfered with your lovely date night with Henry. And you helped so much.'

Nadia waved that away. 'Coming was nothing. Of course I came. It was an emergency.'

'Yes. But you were both wonderful.' Bella touched her hand. 'I knew I could rely on you when I needed you most.'

'You were so calm.' Nadia shook her head. She'd been terrified for her sister. 'It's always been like that. You calm. Me lost.'

Bella smiled, but the smile was unexpectedly shaky. 'Not always. I wasn't calm inside. I could have lost my baby, Nadia. I made the decision not to call the ambulance and hand myself over to people I didn't know. I believed I didn't have time to leave home. I could have got that wrong.'

'But you didn't get it wrong.'

'No. I risked that Ivy was safer fast birthing here than dangerously en route in a cramped ambulance in traffic, but I'm still working through the panic about that. And I don't think Simon is much better.'

Nadia stared. She'd had no idea that her sister ever had doubts about her decisions. 'Bella, I didn't see any of that. Just you, knowing exactly

what you needed to do. I think you're amazing.'
She added, almost to herself, 'And I was useless.'

Bella smiled at her. 'You were perfect. I remember your determination to do everything
Henry asked. You calmed me by doing all the
things I couldn't do and wanted to. So—' here
her sister took her hand '—thank you.'

Good grief, she'd followed orders. But her
grandmother's training kicked in, despite not
being convinced she deserved it. *Always acknowl-
edge a compliment.* 'Well, thank you. You're welcome.'

But Bella wasn't finished. 'And thank you for
feeding Simon dinner and staying to let him de-
brief. He was shocked as well, you know. Poor
darling. Very scary for him.'

Nadia couldn't imagine big, calm Simon
shocked at anything, but she nodded.

'Anyway—' Bella shook her head on something she decided not to say '—we certainly im-
pacted on your date night.'

The dinner, anyway. The rest had progressed,
and boy had it progressed. She still didn't know
what to feel about regretting that. Now wasn't the
time to go there.

'That's fine.'

Bella tilted her head. 'Something's not fine.'
Her brow creased. 'Simon said you and Henry
went home with a bottle of wine and two smiles.
Did you go back to his apartment?'

She didn't want to do this. Not today. But Bella would drag it out of her. Nadia knew her sister's gentle but implacable persuasion.

'Yes, dear. We went back to his place.'

Bella sat forward, interested and thankfully side-tracked. 'Oh. How does it look? I'm curious to know.'

Nadia almost smiled, relieved for the respite. Bella had lived there four years. Of course she wanted to know what her old apartment looked like now.

Furnishings, she could describe. 'Totally different, very blue and white. Masculine but welcoming. He certainly has the knack for creating a relaxing space.'

'I think Henry has a knack for a lot of things,' Bella said softly then waved that away. 'Good on Henry.' She sat back. Fixed her gaze on Nadia's face. 'So, how was it? And what's happened to destroy it?'

Bella had not asked that. 'How was what?' Nadia squirmed just a little.

'Ah.' Bella shifted Ivy's weight on her lap and sat back. 'So…you stayed the night?'

And how could she tell that just by looking at her? Nadia was pretty sure she hadn't been blushing before her sister said that, but she certainly was now. Darn it.

Really no use in holding back. 'It was wonderful, amazing. Beautiful.' Then it came out in a rush. 'But it's all ruined now.'

Bella's face took on that softer, big sis, loving concern. 'What's ruined, darling?'

And that, there, was the problem in a nutshell. And how did she explain?

'Everything. Stopping just when I thought it might work. I'm too close to falling in love with a man just like our father.'

She'd said it. Oh, my, she'd said it. For a few seconds there it had felt as if she'd let it out, but then all the terror rushed back as if in a vacuum she couldn't escape.

'Yes?'

She thought of her daughter's face under the silver crown, her tears. 'He promised to come with us this afternoon, didn't arrive, and then called and cancelled from work. Katie cried when he let us down again.' She forced her breathing to slow. 'Katie cried. Like we did with Dad.'

Bella looked towards the back yard, where the happy squeals of children playing could be heard. 'Katie seems fine now.'

'Well, she wasn't.' Nadia crossed her arms.

Bella patted her baby's bottom. 'Did you cry?'

'No.' Nadia shook her head. As if. 'I was too darned angry.'

'Because he couldn't leave work?' Her sister's voice came softly.

Nadia threw up her hands. 'Because he promised.' How had she ended up on the back foot when it was all Henry's fault?

Bella laughed. 'Well, isn't he a silly man. Promising what he couldn't give. Did you pressure him for that?'

Nadia's racing mind stopped. Thought. Mulled over that. No. He shouldn't have promised. Couldn't promise. Had she forced him to that? No. Had she made him? Because what if he'd come to her and a child had died?

'Oh, heavens above.' She put her face in her hands. 'And I think I love him. Which terrifies me.' And maybe she'd blown all this out of proportion because of that. *Hell's bells.*

Bella sat quietly for a few minutes and let her think. She did that well. Always had. Then she said, 'What terrifies you the most? That he won't be there for you?'

She hated the thought of that, but it didn't terrify her. She'd been on her own for years. Which was an eye-opener. So why was she so hot under the collar?

And then… Finally, Nadia saw it. Felt it. The fear grew from the bottom of her soul and exploded into comprehension. 'What if something happened to Henry? What if he died too?'

Before Bella could say anything, Nadia whispered, 'I had no idea that was it.' She pressed her chest where the angst had gathered like a huge, hot brick. 'Henry's such a wonderful man. What if I lost him?' She closed her eyes. That was what she was terrified of. *Oh, my heaven.*

She whispered, as it all came clear, 'I suspect I would fall deeper and deeper in love because Henry's not a boy to leave me for his toys.'

'No. He's not a boy. Not at all.' Her sister smiled softly. 'Though all men are boys inside somewhere.'

Nadia blinked back sudden tears. She'd seen the boy inside Henry once. Had wanted to nurture that child. Had even imagined briefly what Henry's son might look like.

She murmured, 'When Alex died, I lost my dream of the life I imagined with him.' She couldn't think of another word for dream. That was what it had been. Just the thought gave her chills. 'If that happened with Henry...' And she had had secret dreams. She saw that now. The three of them at a theme park, like Henry had said. Walks on the beach. Maybe even a baby together. She hadn't realised she'd been dreaming as well as fighting against it.

And she could lose it all if he died. Terror shimmied inside her.

'I don't think I could pick myself up again, Bella. I'm not even game to think about that. I couldn't watch Katie go through the pain that I know will never leave her if something happened to him—because pain doesn't leave when you lose someone.'

Bella nodded with understanding. 'We saw that with Dad.'

Nadia blinked. 'What?'

'He was never the same after our mother died. And that fear is understandable,' Bella said quietly. 'There was a cost when Alex died. I get you don't want to go there again…can't imagine being back in that void. Anyone could understand that.'

Ivy squirmed and Bella lifted the infant until she was over her shoulder and gently patted her back. 'You and Simon are very similar in your fears.'

'You mean because Simon lost his wife?' Because he'd been a widower, like she was a widow? She'd forgotten that. But when Bella and Simon had fallen in love there'd been so much going on.

She'd been struggling. Leaning on Bella. Alex had been gone suddenly. Debts, she'd nearly died, her baby had been premature, and dear Gran had been unconscious.

It was as if Bella heard all the thoughts as they skipped through her mind. 'Yes. It wasn't a good time. Do you remember me telling you anything about how Simon lost his first wife?'

Nadia frowned. 'Maybe. Yes.'

'His wife and his baby both died,' Bella said softly. 'Amniotic fluid embolism while he was on call.'

'He was called back to the hospital when it happened?' She thought of the last twenty-four hours for Simon and Bella. 'Like yesterday, when he wasn't here?' Nadia thought that through and felt a chill rise the hairs on her arms. 'He was called out yesterday as well?'

Bella's eyes were shiny with emotion. 'Yes. And my waters broke and the cord came first.'

'Oh... And you could have...' Nadia's voice trailed off. Her sister and Simon could have lost their baby. While Simon wasn't here.

Bella nodded. 'Which is what knocked Simon so much, because again he was at work and I needed him.'

'Oh, my heaven...' Nadia breathed. It seemed even the best relationships had challenges. And terrifying moments.

Bella wasn't finished. 'Like you, when Simon first met me, he was afraid of risking his heart again. So he fought against his attraction. Denied the obvious pull we had to each other. He pushed me away. Firmly. Like you're doing to Henry.'

Her sister leaned forward. 'Nadia, I think Henry loves you. And you say you might love him. You have to decide if you'll risk never knowing that joy—because the chance of finding your life partner is worth all the risks—and the joy is why.'

Nadia heard the words. Felt them sink into her heart like a new colour ink into chalk. A concept that made sense of a new beginning. Of taking risks. Of managing disappointments. For the joy that she did find in Henry's company.

Yes, Henry was colour. Light. Joy. Henry was new beginnings. Henry loved her, loved Katie, and last night, wrapped in his arms, she knew she loved him. The reality was that if she kept pushing him away she would lose him just as surely as if she denied what they had. A different type of fear sank in.

CHAPTER TWENTY-FIVE

Henry

HENRY WISHED HE'D never mentioned theme parks to Nadia because he thought he might just have jinxed himself. This relationship, rollercoaster, ride of his life with Nadia and Katie was tearing him apart.

The day had started with such a high after the night with Nadia in his arms, Henry buzzed, as if someone had pressed him into one of those recharging ports for electric cars. But he suspected he was running on borrowed time with the little sleep he'd had in the last few days.

Work had been huge this week and last night with Nadia had been overwhelmingly amazing but not restful.

This morning, Nadia hadn't done anything to alleviate his unease. One minute she was wild and wanton and the next she wanted to get away and the panic had come and gone in her blue eyes like a flashing light. He'd seen it. Tried to ignore it because he'd had to leave.

He understood they'd probably progressed faster than they should have, and if his own impatience cost him his chance he would never forgive himself.

Plus, he couldn't shake a sense of foreboding after that last phone call, when she'd said she understood but there had been finality in her tone...

He'd been stupid to promise he'd go with them. His brain had said he'd just let her down at lunch and the ward had seemed sorted. Until Emergency had phoned. He'd wanted to see Katie's eyes when she saw Bella's baby. But he'd let them down again.

Now that he could finally leave, he hadn't eaten and he needed to sleep in case he was called out tonight.

He could make some fast eggs for the protein but wondered if Nadia was home. Maybe they would be back from Bella's, and he wanted to apologise in person.

When he knocked on her door he half expected Katie to answer the tap of his knuckles, but no one came. He tried again, listening to hear the sounds of movement and voices, but nothing. At least he didn't think they were pretending not to be there.

His disappointment seemed out of proportion to the fact that Nadia had probably gone to see her sister and the new baby instead of waiting around for him. Of course.

And of course she wouldn't mention where she'd gone to him, because why would she? He was nobody.

He'd let her down again. He'd been going to organise more backup. Maybe he should look at trying to stick with just overseeing the children's ward and let someone else take over the paediatric cover in the emergency department.

If he wanted a life outside the hospital.

He wondered if Marco would be interested.

Ah, hell. Exhaustion swamped him. He looked at the stairs that led from Nadia's floor to his apartment so many floors above—he should climb them instead of taking the lift.

For a moment, he rested his head on the handrail post and sank to sit on the cold concrete and closed his eyes.

'Did you go to sleep outside our door?' the little voice said loudly.

Henry's lids flew open. Katie's bright green eyes were right in front of his face. He blinked. Straightened his cricked neck. Licked his dry lips and focused. 'Just for a minute.' But the cold ache in his backside and pain in his neck said otherwise.

He rubbed his neck. 'I might have dozed off.'

'You didn't come with us to see the baby.' Accusing. 'I put my princess dress on for you.'

'No, I had to work.' He winced at the accusing green eyes level with his own. She was wearing a silver crown. 'I like your princess dress very much.

He climbed to his feet. He could hear Nadia coming down the hall from the garage and he pushed the hair out of his eyes and tried to look like he hadn't slept outside her door like a stray dog.

Hopefully, she wouldn't notice his dishevelled appearance.

'Dr Henry was asleep on our stairs,' said Katie loudly and with much glee.

Henry winced and groaned.

Nadia came around the corner and looked him up and down. 'I see that. I think Dr Henry was awake a long time last night and needs to sleep.'

The beautiful woman he'd been dreaming about, maybe not realistically, smiled at him. Which was a good thing. Always.

There was something different about her smile. Something warm and caring, a promise he could almost hope for, and his heart gave an extra thump like the dog's tail he might have grown while he was asleep.

She opened the door and pushed it wide. 'Come in, Dr Henry. Look at you. Have you had anything to eat today?'

He shook his head, and she shook hers admonishingly back. 'I can feed you. Only fair. You're always trying to feed me.'

And suddenly it wasn't so bad he'd been caught napping.

Henry had no idea he loved hot toasted cheese and tomato sandwiches on grain bread so much. He ate four of them. That was eight slices of melted food on bread. As soon as he finished one, Nadia slipped another steaming one onto his plate with a spatula. 'Stop,' he said. 'Stop. I'll get carbohydrate overload.'

She laughed. 'I'm sure you'll burn it off. But I'll stop.' She set down a big mug of incredibly aromatic tomato and herb soup and said, 'Drink the soup as well.'

So he did and felt almost human by the time he'd finished the mug.

He could hear Katie talking to Ernestine in the bath. Ernestine watched, she didn't bath, Nadia had said, but she certainly joined in the conversation, according to Katie's responses. Henry smiled at the thought. He could love a doll.

He hadn't realised he'd been so cold sitting on the step in the dim and chilly hall, but it was the warmth of Nadia's smile as she fussed over him that made him heat on the inside.

She tilted her head at him. 'It's lucky you're a

handsome man, Henry. Even sleep creased and ruffled you're irresistible.'

He was? 'I am?'

'Oh, yes,' she said calmly as she walked back into the kitchen with his empty mug.

He stood, watched her rinse the cup, took several steps towards her and when she acknowledged he was there he slid his arms around her waist.

The scent of her filled his head. He nuzzled her neck. Whispered into her ear, 'I love you. Very much. Will you marry me?'

She leaned into him. Kissed his throat. 'I'm thinking about it.'

He thought about that. He could wait. 'I'll ask you again tomorrow. Wanna make popcorn?'

CHAPTER TWENTY-SIX

The wedding

NADIA HADN'T WANTED a big wedding. She'd had one of those and Alex had said, *'No children allowed.'* But this time she wanted a small family wedding, with little formality and Henry.

Henry just wanted them married and what Nadia wanted stood well by him.

All Katie wanted was to be flower girl.

So they set their wedding stage across the road from Bella and Simon's house on the sandy beach at Bilinga and aimed for fun.

Henry had secured council permission to erect a three-sided wedding marquee on the sandy grass and the finished landscape ended up looking more like a cross between a circus and a children's playground than a wedding reception venue.

Simon and Mr Tierney had moved the trampoline across the road and fenced off an area with play equipment and a shaded, shallow wading pool for later in the warm afternoon. Parents would be able to watch the children playing in front of them while enjoying the smokehouse at the side of the marquee when that came around with the caterers.

The whole front of the marquee lay open to the sparkling afternoon seascape while the sun passed overhead. White tables, blue cutlery from Lulu's restaurant and flowers climbing the poles to the roof made the shady space look pretty and festive. The air was filled with the scent of flowers.

The mix of guests was adults, lots of children, two babies and a few key people from the hospital. Plus Lulu and her boys.

Henry's registrar Amelia and his two residents, plus Nadia's friends from the children's ward were there. As well as Henry's best man, Marco, a ridiculously handsome Italian with the sexiest accent, who had arrived from London and became enamoured of the Gold Coast and the weather. He completed the assembly.

Marco had taken Nadia up on her offer of renting him the ground floor unit and would be working with Simon and Henry in the paediatric practice for the next year while he sought permanent residency. He'd taken over paediatric emergency admissions. He didn't know it yet, but he was Henry's backup plan for date nights.

Nadia dressed across the road at the Purdy house, with Catherine and Bella as her assistants. They tweaked her strapless pearl-coloured sheath dress until it smoothed over her skin from bodice to her 'something new' silver sandals.

Her hair had been swept up into a tiny silver half-crown with falling golden curls and a tiny veil to float around her shoulders. A gifted and magnificent pearl-drop earring set, more than a hundred years old, was the 'old' and they matched her grandmother's pearl necklace to be the 'borrowed'. On her wrist, she wore an intricate and jewelled 'blue' bracelet, gifted from Henry, who swore the glorious aquamarines were the exact colour of her eyes.

Malachi and Lisandra's two boys, Bastian and Bennett, were the matching pageboys in black suits, looking very similar as twins often did.

And Katie was the prettiest flower girl in the world with her basket and her rose petals to scatter on the sand. And she wore her crown.

'It's time to go,' said her father and Nadia sucked in a breath.

Professor Piers Hargraves looked very distinguished in his grey suit and blue silk tie the same colour as Katie's dress.

Very softly, so nobody else could hear, he said to Nadia, 'You look very like your mother.' His voice held emotion she'd never heard from her austere dad and her eyes misted at the gentleness in his tone. 'You've always looked like your mother,' he said. 'Painfully so. I loved her very much.'

'We lost you when she died, didn't we?' she asked quietly and loving Henry now, as she did, she could see her father in a new light.

Piers closed his eyes. 'I think so. And I'm sorry. But you've grown into a beauty, Nadia, and I'm very proud of you. I wish you a wonderful marriage with this man. I think you've chosen well.'

Nadia's chest tightened and she leaned up and kissed her father's cheek. 'I think so too. Thank you.'

Across the road, Henry waited at the edge of the water with his back to the horizon, listening to the sounds of the waves as they came behind him in the surf. In front of him were the two dozen guests in white chairs they'd spread on each side of the Aegean blue carpet ready for his bride.

She'd be here soon.

Beside him stood Marco. For once, his friend looked serious. 'You're a lucky man, Henry,' he murmured.

Henry smiled. He was. 'I know it.'

He glanced at his friend and caught him studying Amelia with a discerning eye. *Oh, no, you don't.* He cleared his throat until Marco looked back his way. 'And I appreciate you being here for the occasion.'

Marco's eyes gleamed. 'I'll be here for more

than that,' he said, and his gaze drifted left again towards Amelia.

'No, you don't,' Henry pretended to growl. 'I need my registrar.'

Marco laughed but Henry saw a movement across the road and his attention zeroed in.

Ah. She was coming. All other thoughts fled.

On the other side of the pedestrian crossing two figures dressed as school traffic wardens held up stop signs. Henry had to grin. The Tierneys were traffic wardens before they were guests.

The Saturday afternoon cars slowed and stopped.

When it was safe, Isabella Purdy and Catherine Hargraves each held the hand of Henry's new little daughter, Katie, all dressed in blue. She skipped with her basket between them.

After them came Lisandra and Malachi's two boys.

And finally, his love. His future wife. His gorgeous Nadia on the arm of her father, looking like the angel she was.

Henry's heart swelled and he sucked in a breath. Beside him, Marco murmured reverently, *'Bellissima.'*

'She is, indeed,' said Henry. 'My darling love.'

* * * * *

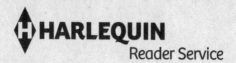
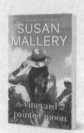
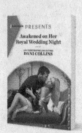
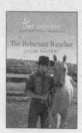
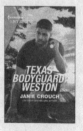